10 Years
Younger
in 10
Weeks

Our Trees

By buying this book you also bought the
right to get a tree planted.

Go to **www.pinetribe.com/planting**
to claim your tree.

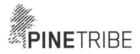

PINETRIBE

Going digital is good for the reader, good for the author and good for the
planet. That's why at Pine Tribe we only deliver digital books and print-on-
demand to minimise waste. But that's just the start of our quest. We plant lots
of trees. We just love trees. Maybe you do too.

10 Years Younger in 10 Weeks

NATURALLY SEXY
FOREVER

THORBJÖRG,
54 YEARS YOUNG

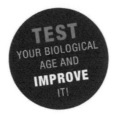

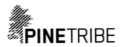

10 years younger in 10 weeks
© Thorbjörg Hafsteinsdottir and Pine Tribe Ltd. 2014

Cover design and typeset: Klahr | Graphic Design
Photographer (cover, cases and of Thorbjörg): Tuala Hjarnø, www.tuala.com
Additional Photos: Line Thit Klein, www.lineklein.dk
Styling: Christina Wedel and Ditte Risted, www.stylemansion.dk
Editors: Julia Hilliard and Kalimaya Krabbe
Translator: Robert Hay, TRANZLATE

1st edition 2014

ISBN: 978-0-9912609-2-8

www.pinetribe.com/thorbjorg

Pine Tribe Ltd.
International House
1 St Katharine's Way
London, E1W 1UN

CONTENTS

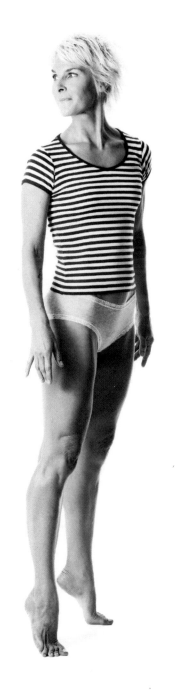

DISCLAIMER

Nutritional benefits may vary from one person to another. The information in this book and its accompanying website is designed to help you make informed choices about your health. It is not tailored to the needs of your specific situation and is not meant to substitute for the advice provided by your own physician or other health professional. The program in the book and website is not intended to cure any medical condition, and if you have one or are taking medication you should consult your doctor before you start this program.

If you have or suspect that you have a medical problem, promptly contact your health care provider.

This book is meant to be inspirational - the Author and Pine Tribe Ltd. cannot be held liable in any way for what is stated or displayed.

For more information see **www.pinetribe.com/thorbjorg/disclaimer**

thank you · thank you · thank you

~~~~~~~~~~

This book is dedicated to the most important women in my life, whom I love unconditionally: my beautiful mother Ingveldur, who is my most important teacher in the art of being ahead of the times; my three beautiful and lovely daughters, Ásta Lea, Ida Björk and Telma Pil, who teach me to be in the present times.

I count myself lucky for being surrounded by wonderful women, who have been with me and supported me on the making of this book. And most importantly, thank you to the thousands of women, who have trusted me and have gone anti-age with me. Well done!

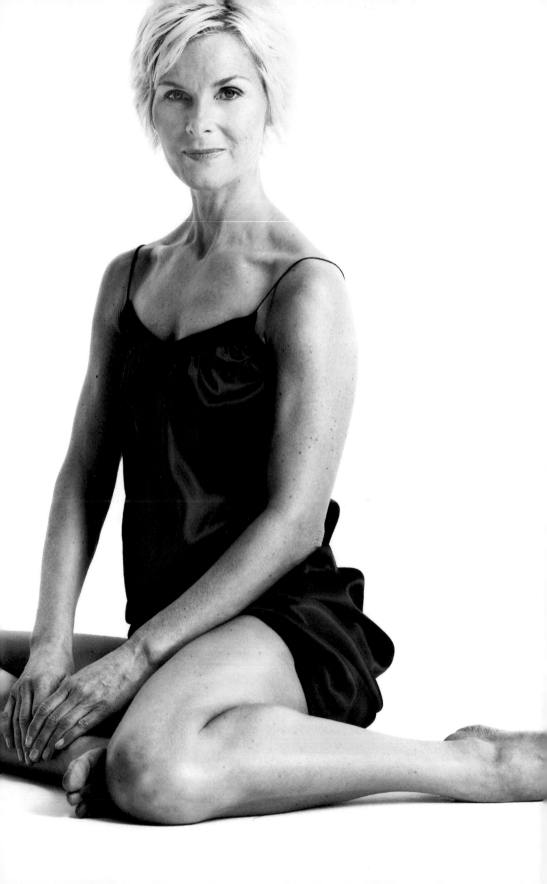

CHAPTER 1

My story can be your story too

~~~~~~

I'll never look old

Author: Thorbjörg from Iceland
Age: 54 years young, mother of three
Profession: nutritionist and nurse with 20 years' experience

It's not every day you hear people praising women in their 40s and 50s for their smooth complexion, sex appeal, unlined faces and youthful bodies. Are you tired of hearing negative talk and gloomy forecasts for life after 40? Does it make you nervous to think about your body going into decline, your skin beginning to sag, and your buttocks becoming as droopy as the corners of your mouth – and getting worse as the years go by? Does it make you sad to think that good-looking men will no longer give you the once-over? Do you worry about dryness, hot flushes and mood swings, which will supposedly supplant your bodily juices, vigour and sex drive? This only happens if you don't get the right vitamins, minerals, oils and the other substances that you need to preserve your youthfulness right to the end. Sugar, bad food, stress and passivity make you old before your time. The good news is that the solution is right here in your hands. You no longer have to think about 40+ as the age of repair. This is the beginning of your sexy years.

I'm doing fine

I'm 54 years old. My skin is firm. I can still get young guys to give me the eye, I'm constantly being complimented on my firm skin, and I wear tight jeans. I don't suffer from hot flushes, dryness or inexplicable weepiness, and I don't have sagging skin, wrinkles, cellulite or love handles all over the place. We don't normally say things like this about ourselves, but I presume you bought this book to learn my secrets! I know that I'll still be sexy when I'm 60 and when I'm 70. I'm not going to look old because I make an effort to look after my body, and I can teach you how to make this possible. I'd like to tell you why my method is worth copying.

I make a living by making women beautiful, healthy and in love with themselves, but I was also an unhealthy sugar junkie when I was younger. I felt terrible because of the food I ate. I left my home in Iceland and took a job as a maid at a Danish hotel. I don't remember anything from that period apart from all the food I ate. I even gulped down the Danish pastries left on the guests' breakfast trays.

Not only do I have personal experience, but I also have a track record of 25 years' experience working professionally with the kinds of food and additives that actually make you older - perhaps even older than your age. I've also got as many years' experience in slowing down the ageing process and turning back the clock. Those of my friends who knew me 20 years ago say I look younger now. I look forward to hearing your friends say the same thing about you in a couple of years.

Be responsible for your age and beauty

Your body is a wonderful working partner if you treat it well. You can change the expression of your genes, your enzymes, free radicals and all those invisible mechanisms inside you that make you look wrinkled, saggy, sick and tired. With the right way of eating, thinking and living, and by using the right creams, you can become young, firm and beautiful again.

14

I'm sure you would like to be healthy, strong and full of energy and optimism. Perhaps you've had enough of being tired, constipated, dry, bad-tempered and frustrated about what you see in the mirror every morning. Perhaps you'd like to get rid of those extra pounds, that pale sallow skin tone, your sagging skin and all-too-plentiful wrinkles. Or perhaps you feel all right and are basically content with yourself, your health and your looks. You just know that you're ageing. You know that now is the time to invest in the years ahead.

You've come to the right woman. In the coming weeks, we'll change your life. I'll invite you to write a diary, test yourself, and eat hormone-friendly, rejuvenating beauty food and supplements. I'll encourage you to use the only natural anti-ageing products that work and to change your biochemistry. I'll make it possible for you to change your habits and your hormones so that you can personally experience the relationship between your weight, your blood sugar and your energy. The change you will experience will be visible in the mirror in 10 weeks. So remember to take a photo before you begin and place it in your book right away. Welcome to the journey of your life. Travel 10 years back in time to a state that will change you forever.

How to use this book

The intensity of the programme depends on your biological age. The more gentle you've been with your body and mind, the easier the programme will be. There are some chapters that healthier women will be able to skip.

If you've been eating, living, thinking and drinking inappropriately for many years, I'll need to lead you by the hand all the way through the 10 weeks. Once we've done that, you'll know how to use this book, or perhaps I should say, how hard you'll have to work.

Test yourself

I've seen women of 20 with bodies like 50-year-olds. I've met 4-year-old children on their way towards premature ageing because of their lifestyle. And I've met 60-year-old women who were younger both inside and out than their children and grandchildren. You can't see what's going on inside you. That's why your first step is to take the test in chapter 2: *test yourself: how old is your body?*

This book is packed full of important information that will make it easier for you to make the decision to change your life. Throughout the book you will find short tests, which include warning signs to watch out for. The tests will ask you about your digestion, skin, stress levels, diet, and so on. If you find that several of the warning signs apply to you, you'll know you should stop and read about what is causing your symptoms.

My hope is that this background knowledge will inspire and motivate you.

Thorbjörg's daily steps towards eternal youth
– make a couple of them your own or adopt the whole package

1. I splash cold water in my face.
2. I drink a big glass of chilled water.
3. I take my herbal hormone-friendly supplements.
4. I do my push-ups, sit-ups and floor exercises.
5. I mix my morning shake and plan my day while listening to soothing music.
6. I scrub my skin with a soft brush and apply my favourite skin products.
7. Each morning I prepare a packed lunch, snacks and food supplements for the day.
8. I take two five-minute breaks at work each day to empty my head of thoughts.
9. I go to yoga classes or jog every second day – for me, late afternoon is the best time.
10. I make sure I get between seven and eight hours of quality sleep every night.

CHAPTER 2

Test yourself:
How old is your body?

~~~~~~~~

What you eat and drink can be seen and felt

Warning signs that you are older than your age
- Too many wrinkles (smile lines are OK)
- Sagging skin on your face and body
- Dark circles under your eyes
- Bags under your eyes
- White spots on your nails or brittle nails
- Dry skin and dry mucous membranes
- Excess weight or obesity
- Fatigue
- Sallow skin colour
- The whites of your eyes are yellowish
- Liver spots or brown spots on your hands and face
- Double chin
- Dry hair, brittle hair or hair loss

Hidden, dangerous signs of ageing
- Tired organs
- Poor immune system
- Hormone imbalance

- Long and difficult lead-up to menopause
- Difficult menopause
- Blood sugar problems
- Insulin resistance
- Stress
- PCOS (polycystic ovary syndrome, often accompanied by infertility)
- Reduced sex drive
- Poor digestion or constipation

Test your biological age

Your chronological age is one thing - that is, how many years you've lived since you were born. Your biological age is something else altogether. Just how old is your physical body? How old and worn, or how young and "fresh" is it?

Modern food and lifestyle, stress and lack of exercise wear your body down. Even at 20, you can have the body of a 40-year-old. Conversely, you can be 85 with a body as fresh as that of a 60-year-old.

Now for the good news

To say that old age is synonymous with a high risk of illnesses such as osteoporosis, cardiovascular problems, dementia, cancer, rheumatoid arthritis and poor digestion is rubbish. It makes sense in industrialised societies, but only because people eat and live in a way that causes their bodies to break down before their time. For people in some ethnic groups, whose lives and eating habits are healthier than ours, age is not synonymous with serious decay, just as only 20 years ago Japanese women who lived a traditional lifestyle didn't suffer from osteoporosis, even after the menopause. They also avoided all our side effects of menopause – increased risk of cardiovascular disease, breast cancer, hot flushes and dementia. They had, and many of them still have, a low biological age because they give their body what it needs.

Are you ready for the vital truth about your age? Take the test with a smile, knowing that you'll soon be able to do something about it.

Take it as valuable knowledge if you find out if your age is high be-cause you wear your body down more than it deserves. Or see if you score a low biological age as a reward for eating healthy food and having a good lifestyle. This questionnaire will give you an idea of your biological age. It can't be compared with medical examinations, but it can help you take stock, and is the perfect start to your new life. *Inspired by material by Dr David Wickenheiser, Burnaby, BC, Canada.*

You can also test your biological age online.
Go to **www.pinetribe.com/thorbjorg/age-test**

Section A – chronological age

What is your chronological age?

Section B – eating habits

How often do you eat fried or grilled food?	Often = 4
	Once a day = 3
	A couple of times a week = 2
	Once a week = 1
	Very rarely = -2
How often do you eat virgin oils that have NOT been heated or used for frying (e.g. flaxseed oil or extra virgin olive oil)?	Never = 2
	Once a week = 1
	Daily = 0
	2+ times daily = -2
How many portions of vegetables and berries do you eat per day (1 portion = 1 piece, 100 g or 4oz)?	I almost never eat any = 3
	A couple of times a week = 2
	1 portion per day = 1
	3 portions per day = -1
	5+ portions daily = -2
How often do you eat wholegrain products and/or fibres (e.g. whole-meal flour, sunflower seeds, brown/wild rice, flaxseed, rye bread with seeds or oats)?	Very rarely = 3
	Once a week = 2
	A couple of times a week = 1
	Often = - 2

How many glasses of water do you drink per day? (Coffee, black tea, soft drinks and alcohol do NOT count).	I rarely drink water = 3
	1 glass per day = 2
	4 glasses per day = 1
	8 glasses per day = 0
	10+ glasses per day = -2
How often do you consume sugar, foods containing added sugar, sweets or candy, soft drinks, or white flour?	3+ times daily = 3
	Once a day = 2
	A couple of times a week = 1
	Almost never -3
How many standard units of alcohol do you drink per week?	12+ drinks per week = 3
	8 drinks per week = 2
	4 drinks per week = 1
	2 drinks per week = 0
	Almost never drink = -1
How often do you sprinkle salt on your food?	On all my food = 2
	Daily = 1
	A couple of times a week = 0
	Once a month = 0
	Almost never = -1
Total score, section B	

Section C – food supplements

How often do you take multivitamins or mineral supplements?	Almost never = 2
	Once a week = 1
	A couple of times a week = 0
	Every day = -1
How often do you take antioxidants (e.g. vitamin C, natural vitamin E, selenium, grape seed extract or green tea extract)?	Almost never = 3
	Once a week = 2
	A couple of times a week = 1
	Daily = -2
Total score, section C	

Section D – daily habits and activities

How often do you exercise / are you physically active (30 minutes of continuous physical activity)?	Almost never = 3
	Once a week = 2
	3–4 times a week = -2
	5+ times a week = -3
How often do you exercise for more than 2 hours at a time? (Score "4", if you never exercise).	Almost every day = 4
	50% of the time = 2
	Almost never = 0
How often do you sleep well and wake up well rested?	Rarely = 3
	Sometimes = 2
	Most of the time = 0
	Always = -1
How often do you pass stools?	Once a week = 4
	Once every four days = 3
	Once every second day = 2
	Daily = -1
	2+ times daily = -2
Total score, section D	

Section E – medical background

Do any of the following diseases run in your family: cancer, diabetes, cardiovascular disease, depression, obesity/excess weight, liver problems/diseases, high cholesterol or high blood pressure?	Two or more of these = 1
	One of these = 0
	None of these = -1
Have you ever suffered from any of the following health problems: cancer, diabetes, cardiovascular disease, depression, obesity/excess weight, liver problems/diseases, high cholesterol or high blood pressure?	Two or more of these = 3
	One of these = 2
	None of these = -2

How often do you suffer from one or more of the following: headache, fever, sore throat, sore muscles not due to exercise, cold or flu, itching/rash or swelling?	Every day = 4
	Every week = 3
	Every month = 2
	Rarely = 0
Are you ever exposed to environmental toxins or similar? (For example from car mechanic workshops, at the hairdresser, during beauty treatments.)	Every day = 4
	Every week = 3
	Every month = 2
	Rarely = 0
Do you have any amalgam fillings in your teeth?	3+ fillings = 4
	2 fillings = 3
	1 filling = 2
	No fillings = 0
Total score, section E	

Section F – stress factors and loads

How many large meals do you eat per day? (Snacks do NOT count).	None = 3
	4+ per day = 3
	3 per day = 0
	2 per day = 1
	1 per day = 2
How much time do you spend in front of electronic equipment at work and/or at home (e.g. in front of the television or the computer, or near high voltage power lines)?	8+ hours per day = 3
	6+ hours per day = 2
	A couple of hours per day = 1
	I rarely spend any time = 0
How often do you smoke or are you exposed to passive smoking?	Most of the day = 4
	A couple of times per day = 3
	A couple of times per week = 1
	Very rarely = -1
How often do you take recreational drugs?	Daily = 4
	Once a week = 3
	Once a month = 1
	Never = 0

How often do you drive in heavy traffic?	I constantly drive as part of my work = 3
	3+ hours daily = 2
	1–2 hours daily = 1
	Almost never = -1
How much do you feel stressed at work or at home?	A great deal = 4
	Quite a lot = 3
	A moderate amount = 2
	A little = 1
	Almost none = -2
Total score, section F	

Calculate your biological age

Section B – eating habits	
Section C – food supplements	
Section D – daily habits and activities	
Section E – medical background	
Section F – stress factors and loads	
Total score for sections B, C, D, E and F	
Your biological age *Add the total score from sections B, C, D, E and F to your chronological age.*	

23

Your biological age	Comments
Minus 11 years or less (your biological age is 11 or more years less than your chronological age).	Your health is probably as good as it can be and the prospects that it will remain like that are really good. You make the right choices when it comes to taking care of yourself. Continue with what you're doing! Some of my advice may however be of use to you, and you would benefit from the detox programme once a year.
Minus 1–10 years (your biological age is 1–10 years less than your chronological age).	Your health is probably really good, and the prospects that it will remain that way are good. Focus on maintaining your healthy lifestyle with good food, stress management/control, exercise and so on. Look at how much grain you are eating. The detox programme once a year would be good for you.
Your biological age equals your chronological age.	Your health is probably good and the prospects that it will remain like that are reasonable. However, if you want optimum health and maximum energy, you'll have to make some changes. The right food can do wonders. And look into exercise habits. You might want to make some changes.
Plus 1–10 years (your biological age is 1–10 years more than your chronological age).	Your health is probably OK, but if you continue in the same way, you'll further increase your biological age. The long-term consequences are an increased risk of disease and health problems. Better eating habits and an improved lifestyle would make a huge difference. Follow the 10 years younger programme.
Plus 11–20 years (your biological age is 11–20 years more than your chronological age).	Your health is probably average for the Western world. You run a moderate risk of experiencing health problems and disease within the next five years. Your energy has probably already begun to diminish and it'll get worse with time. Better eating habits and an improved lifestyle are essential and would make a huge difference. You are in a very good place. You have everything to gain and once you get started you will experience positive effects quite quickly.
Plus 21 years or more (your biological age is 21+ years more than your chronological age).	Your health isn't good and there's a great risk that you'll experience health problems or disease within the next couple of years, if you are not already. Your energy levels and wellbeing will decline considerably over the next couple of years, if this hasn't already happened. A marked change in eating habits and lifestyle is required right now. Your stress levels must be reduced. The 10 years younger programme is designed for you! Improving your diet and exercise habits is an excellent way to reduce stress, increase energy levels and improve your health.

How to use the result

You're your age or younger

Congratulations. Go straight to the recipes and super products.

You don't need detox weeks 5, 6 and 7, but you may want to include them for the experience.

You're 1–5 years older than your birth certificate

Follow the programme up to week 5.

You're close to 10 years older or more

Follow the entire programme.

Welcome to the ten most exquisite weeks of your new life

Each week is filled with exciting tasks. You're bound to continue your new routines once you've experienced how much you change, so don't be discouraged. Sugar weaning, for instance, only takes place during week 2. You'll reap the benefits in the form of beautiful skin, excellent mood, and a sense of wellbeing that continues throughout the programme – and for the rest of your life – with your new, sugar-free lifestyle.

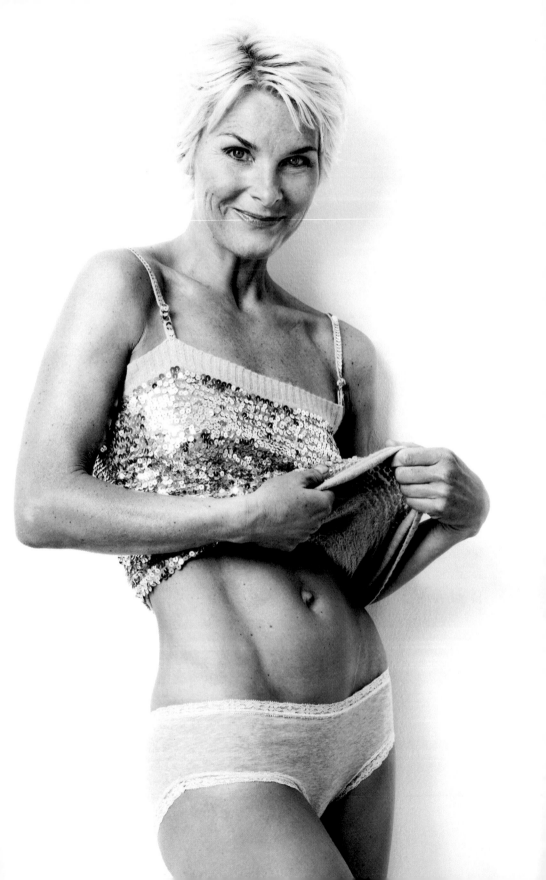

Aware and 100% ready

In 10 weeks you'll have forgotten what you look like now

This week you're going to

document your condition so that in 10 weeks – when everything has changed – you can see and remember what it was like to be you. This week, you'll start writing an anti-ageing diary. There is space for your comments at the beginning of each week's programme. This will become your main tool to maintain good habits and motivate yourself to continue.

You'll need

two good photos – one of your face and one of your body – taken within the last month.

NOTES

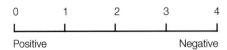

0   1   2   3   4

Positive   Negative

Each week you'll also need to write down what you have for breakfast, lunch and dinner every day. Don't forget to make a note of your snacks.

You can also see and fill out the table online at www.pinetribe.com/thorbjorg/my-charts

	Monday	Tuesday	Wednesday	Thursday	Friday	Saturday	Sunday
Energy 0–4 (describe)							
Digestion 0–4							
Bloating 0–4							
Weight							
Oedemas/swellings 0–4							
Headache 0–4							
Joint pain 0–4							
Muscle pains 0–4							
Bags/dark circles under your eyes/puffy eyelids 0–4							
Nose that runs/is congested 0–4							
Mucous in your airways 0–4							
Rash/eczema 0–4							
Dry skin 0–4							
Concentration 0–4							
Sugar cravings 0–4							
Mental state 0–4							
Feeling low 0–4							
Hormonal problems 0–4							
Irregular periods 0–4							
Hot flushes 0–4							
PMS 0–4							
PCOS 0–4							
Quality of sleep 0–4							
Exercise							

Warning signs of free radicals

- Stress
- High blood pressure
- Heart disease
- Cancer
- Inflammation
- Pain such as joint pain and arthritis
- Type 1 or type 2 diabetes
- Wrinkles and sagging skin
- Eczema and other skin disorder symptoms
- Alzheimer's
- Excess weight or obesity
- Chronic syndromes such as fibromyalgia, which involves muscle pains, fatigue, sleep disturbance and often depression

Free radicals steal your years

Why give your amazing body a load of junk that makes it less beautiful and less pleasant to live in? Know your body's worst enemies and avoid them.

- Environmental toxins and poisons, smoke, pollution, substances alien to your body, heavy metals, chemicals in food and over-processed food
- Chemicals in skin products, cleaning liquids, detergents and electronic equipment
- Radiation
- Infections
- Viruses
- Bacteria
- Fungi
- Other internally and externally originating stress factors
- Inflammation
- Added sugar
- Lack of proper food and nutrition, vitamins and minerals
- Not enough love, human contact and attention

Putting out the fire damaging your body

Life after 35 should only be lit by the flames of passion. Put out the
fire that burns the candle of your life at both ends. This book is an
extinguisher to put out the fire burning in your body at a cellular level
because of free radicals. All your organs, arteries, tissue, ligaments,
muscles, mucous membranes and brain tissue consist of billions of
cells. If, for instance, the cells of the arteries are subject to the "fire
damage" caused by free radicals, they will become worn and old before their time.

The free radicals ravage:

- **The liver,** and can impair the liver's ability to clear toxins from
  your body. If your liver doesn't detoxify well, the result is oxidative
  stress. This can give you fatigue, acne, wrinkles and rashes.
- **The kidneys,** resulting in water retention and oedemas (swelling).
- **The mitochondria,** which are found in most of our cells. The mitochondria are extremely important. They produce energy, which
  the body needs to work and live, grow, be content and happy, run
  and play. Without good energy production, you end up suffering
  from fatigue, lethargy and early ageing.
- **The digestive system,** causing uninvited guests to arrive in your
  stomach and intestines. Bacteria, fungi and other infestations
  cause oxidative stress. Your intestines are connected with your
  brain, and your digestion determines your mental wellbeing and
  surplus energy.
- **Joints and ligaments,** when they hurt or are sore and swollen
- **The heart and blood vessels,** causing high blood pressure and
  heart palpitations.
- **The skin, which is our business card.** Wrinkles and sagging skin
  are caused by oxidative damage to the layers of the skin. More
  about skin, skin nourishment and skin care in chapter 11: *beauty:
  attractive skin throughout your life.*

Stay young with antioxidants and other goodies

Whether your cells age naturally or become visibly "used" and aged depends on the loads you expose them to. It also depends on the rate at which this happens. Let me give you an example. Is your life like a pleasant stroll on a mild, sunny day with an organic fruit smoothie in your hand – without stress and additives, preservatives or other chemicals in your daily life? Or is your life full of chemical skin products? Are you all fired up with no water to cool you down – living a stressful life where you rush around with a burger in one hand and a coke in the other? Are you out of breath and hungry, late for the bus that will take you to the next stressful task? It's the difference in speed and the types of loads and damage your cells are exposed to that determine whether your body ages naturally or prematurely. It also depends on the kind of anti-oxidative defence your body can produce. You can mobilise this defence.

Antioxidants that fight free radicals are, among others:
- Manganese (mineral)
- Zinc and copper (trace elements)
- Superoxide dismutasis (SOD = GliSODine) (super antioxidant)
- Glutathione peroxidase (selenium + glutathione (GSH)) (super antioxidant)
- Vitamin C
- Grape seed extract
- Cranberries
- Pomegranates
- Goji berries

Other great things to prevent wrinkles and ageing are:
- Catechins, which are found in green and black tea, red wine, grape seed extract and dark chocolate.
- Beta-carotene, which is found in all yellow, orange and red fruit, vegetables and berries, for example, carrots, sweet potatoes and red peppers.
- Vitamin E (mixed tocopherols), found in wheat germ.

- GSH (glutathione) and sulphur-containing amino acids found in garlic, onions and cabbage.
- Polyphenols, which are found in green vegetables and lettuces such as spinach, parsley, green kale and brussels sprouts.

Food to fight free radicals

Stressed vegetables are healthy vegetables. Stress is good for vegetables, just as a bit of stress is good for your body because it strengthens your defence mechanisms. Broccoli that grows in an unsprayed field, exposed to sunlight all day, unprotected against attacks by beetles and other insects that want to eat it, is exposed to stress. To resist it, the broccoli has to mobilise its own immune defence. This immune defence is the production of substances called phytochemicals. Broccoli that is very dark, bordering on purplish-green, is stressed and very healthy for humans to eat. When we eat it, we strengthen our own anti-oxidative defence against the "enemies" – the free radicals. That is one of the many things that make organically grown crops more interesting.

So to protect your body from free radicals some great foods you should eat are:

- Vitamins C and A and the many other micronutrients that we get via a diet rich in quality vegetables, fruit and berries
- Carrots
- Sweet potatoes
- Tomatoes
- Fish
- Spinach
- Parsley

Supple, beautiful and sugar-free

~~~~~~

Eating sugar is bound to give you sagging skin and wrinkles

This week you're going to
- experience how you can feel several years younger after only a few days.
- pay into your beauty bank, prevent wrinkles and start your fight against sagging skin.

You'll need
- a large rubbish bag for all the sweet things in your kitchen cupboards and fridge that steal years from your beauty bank.
- a morning shake every day (see the recipe section).
- protein noon and evening (you can use the recipes in this book).
- healthy fatty acids from good quality fish oil and flaxseed oil (see www.pinetribe.com/thorbjorg/cod-liver-oil and www.pinetribe. com/thorbjorg/flaxseed-oil for more information).
- food supplements: chromium picolinate (take 200 μg x 3 times daily with food. See www.pinetribe.com/thorbjorg/picolinate)

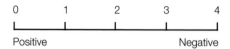

0	1	2	3	4

Positive   Negative

Each week you'll also need to write down what you have for breakfast, lunch and dinner every day. Don't forget to make a note of your snacks.

You can also see and fill out the table online at www.pinetribe.com/thorbjorg/my-charts

	Monday	Tuesday	Wednesday	Thursday	Friday	Saturday	Sunday
Energy 0–4 (describe)							
Digestion 0–4							
Bloating 0–4							
Weight							
Oedemas/swellings 0–4							
Headache 0–4							
Joint pain 0–4							
Muscle pains 0–4							
Bags/dark circles under your eyes/puffy eyelids 0–4							
Nose that runs/is congested 0–4							
Mucous in your airways 0–4							
Rash/eczema 0–4							
Dry skin 0–4							
Concentration 0–4							
Sugar cravings 0–4							
Mental state 0–4							
Feeling low 0–4							
Hormonal problems 0–4							
Irregular periods 0–4							
Hot flushes 0–4							
PMS 0–4							
PCOS 0–4							
Quality of sleep 0–4							
Exercise							

Fatigue

Sagging skin

Wrinkles

Acne or pimples

Dizziness

Difficulty concentrating

Memory loss

Headache

Drama queen behaviour

Mood swings

Aggression

Difficulty sleeping

Hot flushes

Melancholy or depressive thoughts

Sugar dependency

High blood pressure

High BMI (obesity)

Pot belly

No waist

Period problems

Irregular periods

Involuntary infertility

Undesirable hair growth

Bloated stomach

Case study

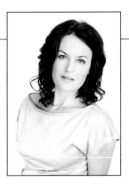

Ninka-Bernadette Mauritson

39 years old, journalist.
Biological age: 30 years.

"I was depressed, tired, absent-minded and had pimples. I looked like a woman of 50 when I was only 33. Now I think I'm beautiful and graceful – and I love the way I look in a bikini. Looking after myself and strengthening my body has become a hobby."

Ninka-Bernadette didn't follow Thorbjörg's anti-ageing programme, but lived in accordance with her principles for about two years – after two years on a detox diet that was too strict.

Before

Previously, I ate a lot of bread, pasta, rice, sugar and cakes and drank sweet drinks. I rarely ate breakfast. I always had sweets, white bread, chips, pasta or anything else that could satisfy my craving for something sweet. Ready-made food, processed meat and food and skin products with heaps of artificial additives, chemicals and E-numbers.

Not a lot of fruit and very few vegetables. I had neither room nor any desire for putting healthy food in my stomach. Occasionally, I pulled myself together and went on a low fat diet. That made me depressed and quick-tempered and I always ended up getting down in the dumps because I invariably succumbed to temptation. Now I know that a stable weight, mind and family life require fats, proteins and heaps of vegetables. And no sugar, white bread or white pasta.

Before, I took no food supplements and got no oil apart from what I used for frying food. I had therefore been struggling with my health

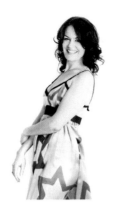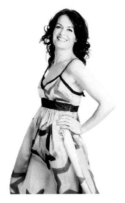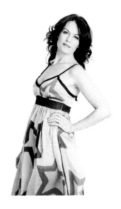

and weight ever since I was 22. I had tried all the diets on the market from low fat products to milkshakes to a strict detox. No matter what diet I was on, my weight went up and down between 68 and 85kg (about 150-190lb).

My shopping habits were typical for the average supermarket shopper – plenty of products with chemicals and additives, ready-made food, spreadable butter and one standard vitamin tablet per day.

My childhood and youth was one long period of despondency and depression right up until I was 33. I tried all sorts of therapists and psychologists, but was depressed most of the time anyway, as well as incredibly tired. I fell asleep during lessons throughout my studies. Later, I fell mentally asleep in my relationships, and in my children's beds when tucking them in. I gave birth to a son with a chromosome defect due to a mutation. I know deep inside that it was a result of the poor food I ate before and during my pregnancy. Now I have transformed his life and mine with Thorbjörg´s help and healthy food and exercise. It saved our lives. Before, I was barely in touch with myself and paid so little attention to myself and my body that I could barely stand other people. I felt that my husband and my children were demanding and sucked all the life out of me.

My fitness was extremely poor. I couldn't run. Climbing stairs made me huff and puff. My sex drive was almost non-existent. I felt frigid. I had large abscess-like pimples on my face and in my groin. My skin was sagging, my face was puffy and I had cellulite. I had a bladder infection once a month, almost always suffered from constipation and often nausea. I remember the nausea as something that always hovered in the background throughout my youth. Now I know it was because of the food I ate.

Now

Today I eat gluten-free, no cows' milk, sugar, white bread or white rice. Plenty of berries and vegetables, and enjoyment. My breakfast is Thorbjörg's recipe; a delicious shake made with frozen fruit, oil and protein powder. Cakes and treats are based on dates, nuts and natural ingredients. I eat whole, unrefined food, organic, no E-numbers and no ruined ingredients. I preferably cook food from scratch.

Food supplements: Thorbjörg's recommended anti-ageing products, vitamins D, C and A, cold-pressed coconut oil, flaxseed oil, fish oil, green tea, selenium, magnesium, calcium and goji juice. To get my stomach going, I take aloe vera or barley grass powder every morning before breakfast.

My weight is stable for the third year in a row: 59–61kg (about 130-135lb).

When I gave up sugar and my cravings disappeared, I was dumbfounded. The depression and fatigue that had hung like a fog over my childhood and youth disappeared. Eating good oils and meat took my sugar cravings away. I recovered my energy and my sex drive. What I thought was a poor family life and a weak psyche was in fact sugar abuse. I'm reminded of this when I occasionally choose to eat sugar on festive occasions (a couple of times a year) – I become aggressive, weepy, depressed and so tired that all I can do is sleep. I thank God for that insight. My mood is stable and I no longer have emotional ups and downs for no reason. Even the jealousy of my youth has disappeared.

I'm in top shape. I run 5km in about 23 minutes. My body is firm and muscular. I love my exercises, which I do at home on the floor (stomach exercises, push-ups and muscle toning exercises). I'm addicted to my daily runs. Before, I used to hate any kind of exercise.

Read more great cases at www.pinetribe.com/thorbjorg/cases

Day 1

Get the rubbish bag out – throw away all the nasties that rob you of your youth

- Sugar: white, brown, soft brown sugar, cane sugar, caster sugar and icing sugar
- Syrup in any form (you can have maple syrup only on special occasions)
- Food with added starch or refined carbohydrates
- Artificial sweeteners in any form (see below)
- High Fructose Corn Syrup (HFCS). Added to numerous different foods: beverages, bread, cake mixes, bars etc. Watch out for it, find it and avoid it!

The following products contain added sugar and/or starch or HFCS: fruit yoghurt, yoghurt drinks, ready-made food like sauces and soups, cake mixes, bread mixes, puddings, tomato sauce, pesto, salad dressings, pasta, potato salad, pies, pasties and sausage rolls, white rice, cakes, biscuits, bread, chips, tinned food, gravadlax salmon, mustard, chutney, baby food, ready-made meals, soft drinks, cordial, sweets, chocolate and much more. Check the list of ingredients. You'll be hard pushed to find ANY food on the shelves in your local supermarket without added sugar, starch or chemical sweeteners.

No more chemical sugar

Your body deserves the best, and artificial sugar is not good enough for you. Many people nevertheless look at "light" products every day, wondering whether to buy them. If I had to choose between plague and cholera, I would also be in doubt. I'm amazed that it's legal at all. Aspartame, also known as Nutra Sweet and containing phenylalanine, has a bad reputation. Aspartame is found in more than 5,000 different food products. Basically, all light or sugar-free products are sweetened with either Aspartame or Sucralose, another infamous and frequently used chemical sweetener.

Aspartame and Sucralose, also known as Splenda, are hidden in a large number of different products: sweets, chocolate, soft drinks, cordials, protein bars, protein powder, cake mixes, desserts, ice cream, smoothies, chewing gum, lozenges, milk products, coffee drinks, vitamin tablets and even baby food.

Aspartame, or E951, has nothing to do with sugar. It's a chemical substance made from aspartic acid, phenylalanine and methanol. Aspartame has a number of serious side effects, 90 of which have been documented and reported to the American Food and Drug Administration (FDA). Some of these are headache, migraine, fatigue and irritation, sleep disturbance and loss of hearing. A Japanese study has added a reduced sperm count to the list.

The problem is that we don't know enough about the long-term effects of artificial sweeteners such as Aspartame and Sucralose. We know that Aspartame is converted to methanol and formaldehyde in the body. That makes it a neurotoxin. You might ask yourself: is that something I want in my body with its potential for nerve damage? Sucralose is a synthetic chemical. In the process of making it, three chlorine molecules are added to a sucrose or sugar molecule. A sucrose molecule is a disaccharide that contains two single sugars bound together; glucose and fructose. The chemical process to make sucralose alters the chemical composition of the sugar. Somehow it is converted to a fructo-galactose molecule which do not occur in nature. Therefore your body does not recognise it nor does it know how to metabolise it.

Watch the film *Sweet Misery*. This documentary tells the story of Aspartame victims with Parkinson's disease and multiple sclerosis, and the frightening story of how the substance was approved for sale at all. Among other things, the former US Secretary of Defence Donald Rumsfeld abused his power to get Aspartame released onto the market. You can watch the film on www.pinetribe.com/thorbjorg/aspartame.

Day 2

Throw away all the nasties that rob you of your youth

You might need a whole roll of black rubbish bags. It's starting to be fun throwing out your old life along with all the things that make you old.

Today, it's time to throw out
- White rice
- Plain wheat flour
- Plain spelt flour
- Plain rye flour
- Plain barley flour
- Plain oat flour

Refined grain products are like food without instructions for use. They are grain products without the germ – and the husks that are full of signal substances and fibres. The body therefore cannot read or understand what it's supposed to do with these plain flours. The more processed and finely ground the products are, the harder it is for the body to use them and to perceive them as anything other than sugar. They also work just like sugar in the body.

Whole grains are a bit easier on the blood sugar than the refined ones, because of the lower glycaemic load. But the starch is still underneath the fibres. And there is also the gluten, which makes many lives miserable. Maybe yours too. You might not know if you are gluten intolerant or not until you have not eaten it in any form for a while. The 10 years younger programme invites you to go for it and try it out. You might be surprised by the wonders it does for you.

41

Days 3–7

Shop your way to sweetness and beauty

Now you need to fill your empty cupboards with nutritious anti-age-ing carbohydrates.

Fill your basket with

- Root vegetables – they contain water-soluble fibres that keep your blood sugar under control
- Sweet potatoes (the normal white potato contains too much starch – eat it every now and then with other vegetables)
- Carrots
- Beetroot
- Celeriac
- Turnips
- Parsnips
- Swedes
- Onions and garlic

Cold, boiled potatoes have a lower glycaemic load than both baked and deep-fried potatoes. A home-made cold potato salad is therefore OK.

Pulses

Pulses also contain some water-soluble fibres that hang on to the "tail" of the blood sugar and hold it back so it doesn't rush ahead, causing a huge sugar load and insulin response. Fortunately, it's almost impossible to get too high an insulin response from eating beans such as:

- Chickpeas
- Kidney beans
- Cannellini beans (the small white ones)
- Butter beans

- Black-eyed beans
- Adzuki beans
- Lentils

Your new sweets

A life without sugar doesn't have to mean a life without anything sugary or sweet. Fortunately, there's plenty you can buy, prepare and eat that will fully meet your need for something sweet without causing havoc with your blood sugar, fat cells in your body or chaos in your immune system. You can enjoy:

- All sorts of fruit – and fruit salad from this book's recipe section.
- Exotic fruit – pomegranate, pineapple, watermelon, melon, mango, pawpaw and passion fruit.
- Berries – both fresh and frozen – strawberries, blueberries, raspberries, boysenberries, blackberries, cranberries, etc.
- Dried fruit – raisins, dates, apricots (without sulphur), figs, cranberries and goji berries.
- Sugar-free cakes based on the recipes in this book.
- Sugar-free sweets based on the recipes in this book.
- Xylitol, which is a sugar alcohol and a natural sugar replacement made from birch bark with a limited effect on your blood sugar. Maltitol and erytrithrol (sukrin) are equally good. Stevia in moderation is alright, but make sure it is derived from all-natural stevia leaves. Go for products sweetened with maltitol, for example good, dark chocolate. Pure dark 85%–95% chocolate, raw chocolate or 100% pure chocolate is a must. And good quality organic honey is ok from time to time.
- Raw honey
- Raw agave nectar

Miscellaneous products without added sugar, such as
- Fruit bars and fruit straps or balls (make your own from the recipes in the back of this book).
- Coconut flakes, coarse and lightly roasted.

- Plain non GMO popcorn.
- Chips/crisps every now and then, but only of a good quality, organic and not made from potatoes. Try chips made from carrots, parsnips and beetroot – they are incredibly delicious.
- Sunflower seeds and pumpkin seeds.
- unsalted peanuts, almonds, cashew nuts, pistachio nuts, walnuts and other delicious nuts.
- Almond butter, peanut butter and cashew nut butter are sweet and delicious. Without added sugar of course!

Instead of white rice and white pasta, buy
- Muesli without gluten and added sugar or honey – dried fruit and nuts are OK.
- Wholemeal spelt pasta in all shapes and sizes, and only eat it a couple of times in a month if you can tolerate gluten
- Wholemeal buckwheat.
- Buckwheat noodles.
- Brown rice, brown rice flakes and brown rice flour.
- Barley, if you can tolerate gluten.
- Quinoa – whole, in flakes or as flour.
- Millet – whole, in flakes or as flour.
- Gluten-free oats.

Grain products to eat in moderation include
- Wholemeal products.
- Wholemeal spelt bread from your local health food shop.
- Homemade wholemeal bread.
- Pumpernickel from the health food shop or your local supermarket.
- Wholemeal rye bread from your health food shop or local supermarket.
- Wholemeal bread – also gluten-free.
- Wholemeal rye crispbread (the organic variety).
- Wholemeal biscuits without added sugar.
- Oats.

44

- Homemade oats and fruit muesli based on the recipes in this book (see Chapter 13).
- Homemade gluten-free muesli.
- Homemade wholemeal spelt rolls based on the recipes in this book (see Chapter 13).
- Whole millet is best, but millet flakes and millet meal are also ok.
- Brown rice – also as brown rice flour.
- Whole barley – also as flour.
- Coarse oats – also rolled.
- Whole buckwheat, buckwheat flakes or flour.
- Quinoa – also as flakes or flour.
- Amaranth.

Why only in moderation?

Although they are full of fibres, husks and healthy fats, all grain products contain starch. This has an effect on your blood sugar and therefore on your insulin levels, weight, skin and body. Grain products should accompany the meal – not play the main role.

Food is described as having a high glycaemic load if it consists of added sugar, added starch, refined starchy grain products, junk food or unhealthy fast food. Food with a high glycaemic load is food of a type, quality and amount that loads your blood sugar and therefore stimulates an insulin response.

Don't eat more than one slice of wholemeal bread or two pieces of crispbread at a time.

Bread-free and grain-free shopping?

For some people, it will be necessary to start eating like a cavewoman (or man), with no grain products at all for a limited period of time, in order to re-establish your blood sugar balance and calm down your insulin response. This especially applies to those of you who are many years older than your chronological age according to my test at the beginning of this book. You may find that the cavewoman lifestyle suits you so well, and your body loves you so much, that you will stay that way for the rest of your life!

Instead of ice cream

Enjoy smoothies made from a blend of fruit, berries and spices that enhance sweetness, such as vanilla, cinnamon and cardamom, xylitol and banana. They are completely hormone-friendly, gentle on your blood sugar, suck the life out of the fat monster and stimulate your taste buds. Add healthy oils and proteins. You can find recipes for sweet smoothies in this book's recipe section.

Beauty sugar

Beautiful sugar alcohols that won't make you intoxicated, confused, tired or fat. Xylitol, maltitol, lactitol, erythritrol and sorbitol can sweeten your life without causing a major load on your blood sugar. So can stevia, raw honey and palm sugar. It's actually possible to find excellent dark chocolate sweetened with maltitol.

You're sweet, and that's why you love sweet things

The sweet taste is associated with feelings. The sweet connection is ancient and embedded in our genes. First of all, it's related to the taste of mother's milk – sweet, healthy, satisfying and hopefully associated with warmth, love and a mother's nurturing.

When we were cavewomen, we induced these sweet feelings on rare occasions by collecting berries, sweet root vegetables and honey. Sweet, healthy and used sensibly. We found a beehive and ate all the honey in one go. Our bodies were just as sensible. They converted the sugar we didn't burn for fuel to fat and stored it as energy, which saved lives when the weather was poor or during a hard winter without food. The extra layer of fat was vital. Today, both our feelings and our consumption have taken over. We have no harsh winters or periods of hunger that can help us get rid of the store of energy we acquire daily by gorging on sweet things.

There's sugar in almost all the food we buy at the supermarket. White rice, white bread, white pasta and potatoes are like sugar to the body. Add to that all the pure sugar in the form of ice cream, sweets, sugar, cakes, concentrated fruit juice, fruit yoghurt and soft drinks. It's like eating one beehive a day. It confuses and harms our bodies. It thinks it does us a favour by storing fat and energy for lean times, but the lean times never come. Are you surprised that your clever body hasn't merely adapted physiologically to all this sugar? If so, remember that we have only added sugar to our food for 200 years. That's just a fraction of our evolution, which goes back millions of years.

Sugar gives you rolls of fat and harms your body

Unfortunately, fat cells are self-supporting and need neither insulin nor a means of transport to attach to the blood sugar. They only need sugar. They have a huge mouth, which is always wide open and ready to eat the sugar you put in it. Fat cells are very hungry and greedy. They are also stupid. They argue with your immune system, which answers back by lighting fires (inflammation) in your body. They cause oxidative stress (rust in your body) and make you old before your time. You experience this as swelling, oedema, joint and muscle pain, headache, stiffness, wear and tear and premature ageing.

You become dependent

If your body has to cope with high blood sugar levels for extended periods of time, it can influence your delicate brain. Research proves this. Many of my clients have also experienced it in their own bodies. You can become just as hooked on sugar as on drugs, tobacco or alcohol. The sugar affects the same areas in your brain. Brain cells are able to create their own natural morphine, the so-called endorphins. We benefit from natural endorphin production when having sex or touching, on our daily runs and while undergoing rigorous exercise like marathons or triathlons. They create a brief adrenalin rush and a feeling of happiness. And sometimes they make us want more. Sugar gives us an unnatural, unhealthy state of bliss that, in the long run, causes our body to age.

Are you dependent?

Symptoms of sugar dependency include
- Fatigue
- Difficulty concentrating
- Confusion
- Foggy brain
- A feeling of being inside a bubble
- An abnormal craving for sugar
- An abnormal craving for white bread and cakes
- A desire for alcohol
- Difficulty sleeping
- Melancholy
- Depression
- Digestive problems

Sugar can make you insulin-resistant and old

Sugar dependency and confusion in the brain chemistry are sneaky, in that you risk creating insulin resistance in your cells. This harms not only the brain chemistry, but also the energy production of your cells. Too much insulin in the blood messes up your bodily functions. The fat cells grow and multiply. Result: large fat cells, thicker layers of fat and more rolls of fat. This causes many women to lose their waist. The body becomes masculine to look at, but it is quite possible to be insulin resistant and thin. Type 2 diabetes is one of the world's most common lifestyle diseases and it makes you old before your time. Even children age early because of this disease. I see more and more children right down to the age of three who are diagnosed with type 2 diabetes because of their mother's food and lifestyle before and during their pregnancy. And because of the food they give their toddler, of course.

Symptoms of insulin resistance and syndrome X (a combination of diabetes, high blood pressure and obesity)

- Fatigue
- Sugar dependency
- High blood pressure
- High LDL cholesterol
- Type 2 diabetes
- High level of triglycerides (fat in your bloodstream)
- High BMI (obesity)
- Pot belly
- No waist
- Period problems
- Irregular periods
- Involuntary infertility
- Involuntary hair growth in places where women don't normally have hair

You don't need to have all these symptoms to be insulin resistant, but if you have the first six on the list, you are probably one of the many people who are insulin resistant, or well on your way.

The following is an example of a week's menu which will give you cellulite, high blood pressure, high cholesterol, rolls of fat, fat in your abdominal cavity, extra weight, fatigue, lethargy, a poor sex life, hormonal disturbances, sore joints or arthritis as well as sagging skin and wrinkles. *Bon appétit!*

Meals	Monday	Tuesday	Wednesday	Saturday	Sunday
Breakfast	Strawberry yoghurt with fruit muesli	Three slices of white bread with cheese or jam, coffee with sugar and milk	Fruit yoghurt, coffee with sugar and milk	Breakfast rolls with jam and cheese, café latte with sugar	Brunch with American pancakes, syrup, toast, eggs and bacon, coffee with sugar and milk
Snacks	Oat biscuit with butter and jam	A coke and a chocolate bar	Chocolate biscuits, one cup of coffee with milk and sugar	Nothing	Nothing
Lunch	Tuna and egg sand-wich	Pasta salad with vege-tables	Sandwich (white bread) with cheese and ham, grilled, one Fanta	A rye bread sandwich with prosciutto and brie	Nothing
Snacks	Nothing	Two slices of white bread with jam, coffee with sugar and milk	Nothing	Nothing	Coffee and chocolate cake with whipped cream, coffee with sugar and milk
Dinner	Pasta with meat sauce	Chicken in the ba-sket with oven-roasted potatoes and salad	Fried vege-tables with chicken and white rice	Steak with baked pota-to and salad, mayonnaise dressing and red wine	Pizza with miscellane-ous cheeses, red wine and a coke
Snacks	Chocolate, coffee with sugar and milk	Ice cream and canned fruit in syrup	Ice cream with choco-late sauce	Chocolate cake with whipped cream, brandy and coffee	Popcorn or biscuits, coffee

One of the best experiences of your life is awaiting you – to become sugar-free and energetic, with a clear head, and to stay young for the rest of your life!

Motivational hit list: stay attractive, slim and young without sugar

Three unfortunate consequences of excessive sugar consumption

1. The sugar is converted to fat on your tummy and around your waist. Great love handles and spare tyres. Excess weight makes you old before your time.
2. Sugar is converted in the liver to saturated fat and LDL cholesterol, which is the bad cholesterol. You have probably read that fat was the main cause of bad cholesterol. In reality, sugar is the real villain. High oxidated LDL cholesterol is one of the causes of early ageing.
3. The sugar adheres to cells in your blood - red blood cells, proteins and even to LDL cholesterol particles. I call this formation of "caramels" in the body. They start fires (cause inflammation) and ravage both your body and brain. Imagine sitting an exam or making an important decision in your life with these caramels in your brain. It's not a good idea. Nevertheless, that's what most of us do every day.

The following substances are also sugar

- Dextrose
- Maltodextrin
- Maltose
- Fructose
- Corn syrup
- Glucose syrup

- All other products ending with the word syrup
- Glucose
- Lactose (milk sugar)
- Wheat starch
- Potato starch
- Corn starch
- Modified starch
- Rice starch
- All other forms of starch

You don't need to eat sugar

Instead, eat the following, which are broken down to glucose

- Vegetables, fruit and berries.
- Quinoa, millet, brown rice, buckwheat.
- Beans and lentils.
- Root vegetables such as carrots, beetroot, sweet potatoes and onions.

Breakfast cereals don't make you beautiful

Myth

Breakfast cereals are slimming because they contain plenty of fibre and are low in fat. Therefore they must be healthy.

Facts

You know them from the pictures of slim, beautiful, healthy-looking people on the colourful packaging. If you read the list of ingredients on most breakfast cereals that advertise their slimming effect because of their fibre content, you'll see that each portion contains perhaps 15g of fibre. However, in two portions, you'll generally find more than 40g of pure sugar. And that's just for breakfast. That has nothing to do with health. In addition, your body must cope with the starch, which is like sugar to your body. Avoid all breakfast products with added sugar or starch in any form. Eating them will make you look old.

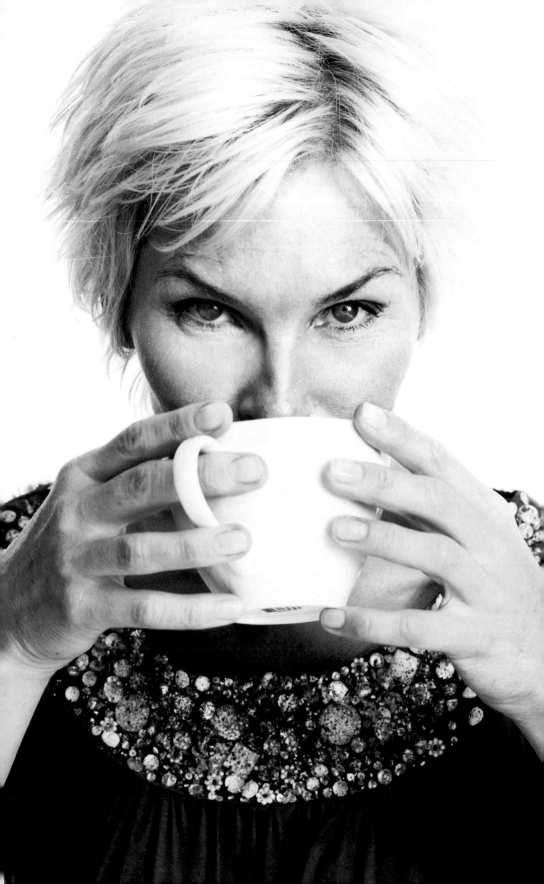

Eat and be young with anti-ageing food

~~~~~~~~

Your second youth begins in the fridge. Eat and be beautiful and 10 years younger

This week you're going to

- read the 10 food commandments, throw things out, buy new raw materials, and begin using the recipes at the back of this book. (See the weekly plan with super anti-ageing food in Chapter 13).

You'll need

- another roll of black rubbish bags.
- a large car for all your new foods.

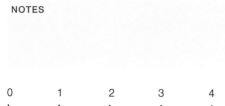

Positive   Negative

Each week you'll also need to write down what you have for breakfast, lunch and dinner every day. Don't forget to make a note of your snacks.

You can also see and fill out the table online at www.pinetribe.com/thorbjorg/my-charts

	Monday	Tuesday	Wednesday	Thursday	Friday	Saturday	Sunday
Energy 0–4 (describe)							
Digestion 0–4							
Bloating 0–4							
Weight							
Oedemas/swellings 0–4							
Headache 0–4							
Joint pain 0–4							
Muscle pains 0–4							
Bags/dark circles under your eyes/puffy eyelids 0–4							
Nose that runs/is congested 0–4							
Mucous in your airways 0–4							
Rash/eczema 0–4							
Dry skin 0–4							
Concentration 0–4							
Sugar cravings 0–4							
Mental state 0–4							
Feeling low 0–4							
Hormonal problems 0–4							
Irregular periods 0–4							
Hot flushes 0–4							
PMS 0–4							
PCOS 0–4							
Quality of sleep 0–4							
Exercise							

Case study

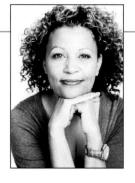

Susan Sogaard

53 years old, founder of the Hard Work fitness
chain and Zenses Fitness.
Biological age: 29 years.

"I shaved more than 20 years off my age in a few weeks. I'll never
return to my old lifestyle."

Before

I suffered from mood swings, stomach aches and bloating. I've always
eaten healthy food, but I had some very persistent extra weight on my
hips. I followed traditional advice about healthy ways to eat. I started
on Thorbjörg's 10 weeks younger anti-ageing course because I wanted
to understand why the way I ate didn't produce the results I wanted.
Of course, I ate sweets every now and then, but I trained and ate low-
fat food. I was healthy, in both my own and other people's opinions.

I hadn't understood the connection between food and mood, and
both my mood and my energy levels were much lower than they are
now after completing the course. The thing that keeps popping up
when I talk to women who live the anti-ageing lifestyle is a past where
they were pessimistic and depressed for no reason. I now know that it
was sugar and the low fat diet that made me feel like that. I felt like
I lived in a fog. I was unable to pay attention when driving. Making
decisions in life was a challenge.

Now

Today, my mood is great and I have plenty of energy. I've shaved
more than 20 years off my age and now know that unhealthy food

and an unhealthy lifestyle cause damage at a cellular level. I eat plenty of cold-pressed healthy fats every day and a lot more vegetables than I did before. I no longer eat sweets and have lost the 5 kilos (about 10lb) I always battled with. I also don't eat white bread, white rice, white pasta or sugar any more. I very rarely drink milk. I've always been in good shape, but now I have the energy and good mood that should accompany a healthy lifestyle. I get good proteins every day in different forms, and take brown rice protein powder in my morning shake. If I'm going out for dinner to a place where I know we're going to have Thai food with white rice, I generally bring my own brown rice. I can feel right away if I haven't had my proteins, greens or oils. My mood drops. My husband also notices it and says: "Let's not make any decisions right now. You need to eat first."

Read more great cases at www.pinetribe.com/thorbjorg/cases

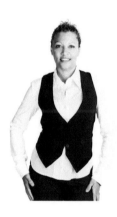 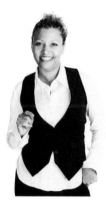 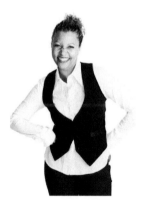

Take a bite out of time

Eat small portions of foods that are gentle to you and your digestion

Eat good quality food containing fibre and healthy fats, berries and little fruits, vegetables and whole grain products.

Eat quality vegetables and other foods that are easy on your digestion
For example:

- Sweet potatoes, asparagus, green peas, celery, berries and beans.
- Wholemeal rye bread with kernels, almonds, sunflower seeds and ground flaxseed.
- If you are gluten intolerant, eat gluten-free wholemeal products: quinoa, buckwheat, millet and rice.

Eat rejuvenating fibres
You can get a lot of fibre by eating fibre-rich food or by taking fibre supplements.

Water-soluble fibres in pulses, beans, root vegetables and fruit are also important for controlling blood sugar levels, so eat:

- Sweet potatoes
- Carrots
- Beetroot
- Turnips, parsnips and celeriac
- Chickpeas
- Kidney beans
- Cannellini beans, black-eyed beans and mung beans

Insoluble fibres are also important, and are contained in wholegrains and vegetables, as well as the husk of pulses and fruit peel, such as:

- Wholemeal rye bread
- Wholemeal spelt bread
- Wholemeal rye crispbread
- Celery
- Asparagus
- Climbing beans
- Sugar peas
- Berries, oranges and apples
- The skins of seeds, nuts and almonds
- Fibre supplements that you can buy in health food shops or at chemists, for example:
  - Guar bean
  - Glucomannan
  - Wheat bran
  - Psyllium husks
  - Flaxseed soaked in water
  - Chia seed soaked in water

Look forward to experiencing your second youth via your digestion. You'll flourish after your anti-ageing cleansing in weeks 5, 6 and 7.

Throw out the youth robbers

- Added sugar.
- Bacteria, fungi and most parasites love sugar! They gorge on it, become big and fat and multiply like mad. Sugar is not good for your intestinal health either.
- That's another reason to completely remove sugar from your life, if you've cheated a bit during the preceding weeks.

- Refined grain products and starch clog your intestines, which doesn't help produce smooth, elastic and healthy mucous membranes that keep you beautiful. Undigested food has a habit of piling up in the folds of your intestinal mucosa, where it solidifies. It can be very difficult for such intestines to react to signals telling them to move, and the peristaltic movements can stop completely. So do your stools and then you become constipated. The longer your stools remain in your system, the more waste products and toxins are released into your blood and body.

- Refresh your memory about refined grain products and products containing starch in Chapter 4.

- Dairy products: milk and cheese. Many people with digestive problems react to dairy products because their intestines have become stressed from unhealthy food, a lack of digestive enzymes and uninvited guests, or because they simply aren't able to tolerate milk.

- Gluten is also a problem for many people who have digestive problems or dysbiosis (a bacterial imbalance in the gut). Gluten intolerance can be the main problem or a secondary problem caused by poor digestion. Gluten is found in wheat, spelt, rye, barley and oats. You can test whether you have gluten intolerance at clinics that practice functional medicine and nutrition. See www.pinetribe.com/thorbjorg/gluten-test

- Yeast in bread and fermented products can also be problematic, as fungi and bacteria love it. The same applies to beer and other alcoholic drinks if the liver is so overloaded that it cannot detoxify alcohol properly. If you react to even small amounts of alcohol and feel intoxicated and awful afterwards, you and your liver are probably working overtime.

- Some people react to lectins in their intestines, either because they lack digestive enzymes, struggle with imbalance of their digestive flora or uninvited guests in the intestines, or simply cannot break down lectins. Lectins are found in fresh (not boiled or baked) tomatoes, in pulses and in all sorts of beans. You can tell if you have this problem if you always get bloated after eating chilli con carne or other food containing beans.

- Make sure you produce a good amount of digestive enzymes. You will be able to do this better if you eat anti-ageing food. Proteins, carbohydrates and fats must be broken down by enzymes produced in the stomach, gall bladder, pancreas and small intestine. Drink water with lemon juice or grape juice before a meal. If necessary, take digestive enzymes as a food supplement together with your food. See www.pinetribe.com/thorbjorg/enzymes for information about purchasing good quality digestive enzymes.

Day 1

Read the following 10 food commandments from Thorbjörg

1. Take care of your body by avoiding added sugar, whether visible, invisible or artificial.
2. If and when you choose to eat bread, eat wholemeal products and whole grains. Your body cannot use refined products.
3. Don't avoid fat. Choose the right fats because they are good for you and slimming.
4. Eat good quality protein.
5. You can eat nuts, almonds, seeds and kernels every day.
6. Eat yourself beautiful with at least 600g (20oz) of organic vegetables, fruit and berries every day.
7. Drink 1½ litres (2½ pints) of water, pure vegetable juice, green tea and herbal tea every day. If you absolutely must have your coffee or alcohol, choose top quality and enjoy it in moderation.
8. Eat regular meals. Never skip your breakfast. Several small meals are the way to go.
9. Eat balanced meals containing healthy fats, quality protein, complete carbohydrates and vegetables. And, of course, make sure as much of your food as possible is organic.
10. Even if you eat excellent food, it's a good idea to take a multi-vitamin/mineral supplement every day. If you want to take other food supplements, consult a healthcare professional first.

Day 2

Emptying – the kitchen cupboards!

From today onwards, have a shake in the morning, and snacks, lunch and dinner based on the recipes in this book. Do this throughout the rest of the programme (and preferably for the rest of your life!). The morning shake equips you for your day's tasks.

Remember

Some women need an extra oil supplement for lunch and at night in addition to what they get in their morning shake. If you get hungry or crave sugar immediately after eating, you're probably one of them. Take 1 tablespoon of cold pressed flaxseed oil or hemp oil in juice after each main meal.

Task

Grab a suitable rubbish bag. Put on your favourite music, and prepare a large jug of water with lemon or a pot of green tea. The task ahead will make you sweat. Begin your war of extermination against food and products that age you.

Throw out

- Food and junk with added sugar or starch, if there's any left after your clean out in week 2.
- Everything that contains white flour – i.e. plain flour, whether normal wheat or durum wheat, spelt, wheat, rye or other types, if you haven't already thrown them out.

- Refined fats. These include all oils that are not both cold-pressed extra virgin and organic. This also applies to coconut oil, which shouldn't be refined either.

Empty the contents into the sink or the toilet bowl and continue to fill your rubbish bag. Remember to drink water! Singing also helps!

- Pesto, pickles and other products containing vegetable oil that is not cold-pressed virgin oil (believe me, they only write it on the product if it is true).
- Breakfast products such as Coco Pops and Nutrigrain, honey-roasted muesli and muesli with added sugar, chocolate or sweetened dried fruit.
- Crispbread, rusks, bread, biscuits (even Tim Tams and shortbread) and cakes.
- Milk chocolate and sweets.
- Sugar and syrup, etc. if anything is left on your shelves after cleaning out in week 2.
- White pasta not made from wholemeal grain.
- White rice.
- Preserved food with added sugar: tomato sauce, etc.
- Chemical sweeteners and hidden sugar if you cheated during the cleaning out in week 2.
- NOTE! If you have wholemeal wheat pasta, wholemeal spelt pasta, brown rice, whether jasmine or basmati, wholemeal rusks (without sugar), wholemeal biscuits (without sugar), oats, barley, millet or buckwheat, then leave it for now.

First aid

Does it feel scary, like it's too much at once? Ask yourself why you're doing it. Write the answers down, for example: "Because I want a better life without added sugar, as I've decided I want more energy, better digestion and to preserve my youthfulness." The food that prevents you from reaching these goals will disappear from your cupboards and your life. You might also want to ask yourself what it will cost you

NOT to get rid of those youth and energy thieves right now. How will you feel three months from now? Two years from now?

It also symbolises a new beginning and freedom from unhealthy food habits and bad decisions. Be kind to yourself. The choices you have made so far were necessary to make you aware that you have to go one step further. That experience is valuable in itself.

Day 3

Emptying – the fridge!

Throw out
- Dairy products that make you old, especially those with added sugar.
- Fruit yoghurt, drinking yoghurt and "light" products.
- If you have organic plain yoghurt, organic plain curd, goat's feta and goat's cheese, then leave it for now.
- Mayonnaise made from refined vegetable oils (those that are not cold-pressed and organic).
- Spreadable butter and margarine.
- Salads with mayonnaise, ready-made salad dressings and dips such as Thousand Island and other products containing additives and refined vegetable oils.
- Desserts, puddings and other ready-made products that contain added sugar and starch.
- Paté, processed meats, etc. that contain milk protein, additives, starch and vegetable oils.

Now you should have room for real food that can communicate with your body and your cells.

Day 4

Emptying – the freezer!

Throw out

- Fast food and other quick solutions that contain bad fat, refined grain, additives, starch or sugar.
- Frozen pizza, doughnuts, cakes and desserts.
- Traditional ice cream with added sugar and bad, refined fats.
- If you have prawns, chicken, fish and red meat, then leave it. You can also keep any frozen vegetables, especially if they are organic. You can buy delicious falafel and bean patties. Leave room for those in your freezer or freezer compartment.

Days 5 and 6

Shop for a new life!

Go to your local supermarket and buy products that contribute to your youthfulness, energy, wrinkle-free skin and mental surplus. I call the basic contents of your new pantry super 20 anti-ageing food. They comprise all the things you will need to mix and combine in many different ways. Make sure you always have these ingredients in your kitchen.

1. Broccoli and kale
2. Green tea
3. Chia seed, flaxseeds, and flax oil
4. Salmon
5. Tofu
6. Tomatoes
7. Sweet potatoes and other root vegetables
8. Almonds and nuts
9. Quinoa
10. Whey protein isolate
11. Blueberries (and other berries), fresh and frozen
12. Watermelon and pomegranate
13. Spinach
14. Lemon
15. Turmeric, ginger and garlic
16. Coconut and coconut oil
17. Mung beans
18. Real butter or ghee from grass fed cows or goats
19. Parsley
20. Organic chicken

However, there is much more than the super-20 foods on the menu. The following is my basic shopping list. Right now, it's important that you let your curiosity and desire to try new things determine the pace, instead of going out shopping for everything at once.

Basic shopping list for your anti-ageing lifestyle
You can also download the whole shoppinglist on
www.pinetribe.com/thorbjorg/basic-shopping-list

Grains
- Whole quinoa
- Brown rice, whole or as flour
- Millet, whole or as flour
- Buckwheat, whole or as flour
- Buckwheat noodles (soba)
- Brown rice noodles

- Oats, coarse
- Wholemeal spelt flour
- Wholemeal spelt pasta
- Wholemeal lasagne sheets
- Barley
- Five grain flake mix
- Wholemeal rye crispbread, or round Swedish crispbread

Nuts and seeds
- Almonds
- Walnuts
- Hazelnuts
- Cashew nuts
- Brazil nuts
- Macadamia nuts
- Pumpkin seeds
- Flaxseeds
- Sesame seeds
- Peanut butter without added sugar, either smooth or crunchy, from your local health food shop
- Almond butter
- Tahini (sesame butter)

Pulses (tinned is alright, provided they are organic)
- Chickpeas
- Mung beans
- Kidney beans
- Lentils, brown or red
- Other beans

Food in tins or jars
- Tuna in brine or olive oil
- Sardines in olive oil
- Mackerel in tomato sauce without added sugar
- Salmon in brine

- Coconut milk
- Organic peeled tomatoes
- Organic tomato sauce (without added sugar)
- Vegetable pâtés
- Tofu
- Gherkins without added sugar (cornichons)
- Sun-dried tomatoes in organic cold-pressed oil
- Mustard without added sugar

Alternative beverages to milk (without added sugar)

- Soy milk
- Rice milk
- Almond milk
- Hazelnut milk
- Hemp milk
- Coconut milk
- Oat milk
- Soya cream
- Almond cream
- Canned coconut milk

Packaged food

- Miso soup, instant. See www.pinetribe.com/thorbjorg/miso
- Organic, instant clear soups
- Miso paste on rice or buckwheat crispbreads

Spices

They must be free of monosodium glutamate (also known as MSG or E621) and be as organic as possible. You can buy certified organic herbs and spices at the supermarket or health food shop. For more information on spices www.pinetribe.com/thorbjorg/spices-msg-free

- Cinnamon powder
- Vanilla pod or powder (not to be confused with vanilla sugar!)
- Liquorice powder. See www.pinetribe.com/thorbjorg/liquorice

- Cardamom
- Rosemary
- Thyme
- Oregano
- Turmeric
- Allspice
- Juniper berries
- Cloves
- Whole coriander seeds
- Garlic
- Organic spice mixes, e.g. Indian or Moroccan
- Black pepper
- Red pepper
- Pepper mixes (e.g. red/pink, black, white, green and allspice)
- Ginger
- Sea salt or rock salt, Himalayan salt
- Bay leaves
- Caraway seeds
- Cumin
- Star anise
- Cayenne pepper
- Wasabi powder

Organic oils
- Cold-pressed extra virgin flaxseed oil
- Cold-pressed extra virgin hemp oil
- Cold-pressed extra virgin olive oil
- Cold-pressed extra virgin coconut oil
- Cold-pressed extra virgin sesame oil
- Cold-pressed extra virgin pumpkin oil

Tea
- Green tea, leaves or teabags
- Green Matcha tea
- Liquorice root
- Other herbal teas. See www.pinetribe.com/thorbjorg/herbal-tea

And now for your sweet tooth
- Xylitol or other similar sugar "alcohols" such as sukrin
- Fruit and nut balls, etc. from your local health shop
- Dates
- Apricots without added sulphur
- Prunes
- Figs
- Raisins
- Cranberries and other dried berries without added sugar
- Fruit rings and slices without added sugar, like apple, banana, mango, pear, peach and pawpaw
- Fruit bars without added sugar
- 85% dark chocolate without added sugar
- Carob chocolate without added sugar
- Raw dark chocolate
- Raw cacao nibs

Fats
- Pure, organic butter
- Ghee

Dairy products
Small amounts of dairy products, if you can tolerate them:
- Organic plain curd cheese
- Organic plain yoghurt
- Goat's feta
- Goat's and sheep's cheese

Vegetables
- Broccoli
- Cauliflower
- Brussels sprouts
- Spring cabbage
- Lettuce
- Spinach

71

- Rocket
- Cos lettuce
- Sweet potatoes
- Carrots
- Beetroot
- Turnips
- Parsnips
- Radishes
- Onions
- Garlic
- Leeks
- Pumpkin
- Zucchini (courgettes)
- Tomatoes
- Red bell peppers
- Leafy greens
- Parsley
- Basil
- Coriander
- Rosemary

Fruit

- All types of fruit
- Berries

Other

- Plain whey protein powder isolate.
  See www.pinetribe.com/thorbjorg/whey
- Rice or pea protein for those who can't tolerate dairy products at all. See www.pinetribe.com/thorbjorg/rice-protein
- Hemp protein powder

Day 7

Prepare delicious anti-ageing food

Make delicious anti-ageing food using the recipes in this book and feel the effects. Take your time eating your food. Eat slowly. Wait five minutes before you have a second helping. You're only just beginning to learn what it means to obtain optimum nutrition, and you will thank yourself for the rest of your life. You've already completed the most important part of your new lifestyle. You've cleaned out your cupboards and made room for super healthy food filled with anti-ageing nutrition for your whole body. Congratulations! Celebrate!

Now the time has come for your body.

Checklist
- My home is my friend – free of all the food that steals my energy and ages me.
- I have my super morning shake under control.
- I have told my family and friends about my decision and asked for their support.
- I'm pleased with my efforts. So far, so good.
- I'm quite proud of myself.

Test your digestion

Do you go to the toilet regularly, and do you get any results? Is it uncomplicated or are your stools hard and lumpy, like goat pellets, or thin and accompanied by the remainders of your last meal?

When I ask my clients about their bowel movements, they brush off the question with comments like: "Everything's normal, no problems there." And then it turns out that they may pass stools only two or three times a week. For them, that is normal! It has always been like that, and they don't know any different. The facts are that you should pass stools 1–3 times daily. It should be more or less odourless, well shaped, brown and preferably float. If you can produce decent stools, you're probably doing well with healthy food rich in fibre. You have a healthy amount of good bacteria in your gut. You also have a healthy amount of digestive enzymes, you drink enough liquid and you exercise regularly. Congratulations! If your visits to the toilet are not quite as regular as that, read this section carefully. A good digestive system is a gift from God. Good health and a healthy body that keeps you young are all about a healthy, well-functioning digestive system and good absorption of nutrients. What do you look like inside?

Medical history		
Have you ever had to take courses of antibiotics that lasted for more than a month, for example, because of acne?	Yes ☐	No ☑
Have you had 10 or more courses of antibiotics of one week's duration since you were born? (A two-week course counts as two courses of antibiotics).	Yes ☐	No ☑
Have you been on the pill or taken any other medication containing female sex hormones for periods of two years or more?	Yes ☑	No ☐
Have you been given prednisolone or other adrenocortical hormones for periods of one month or more?	Yes ☐	No ☑
Have you taken NSAID drugs (painkillers or anti-inflammatory drugs that are not adrenocortical hormones) continuously for periods of six months or more?	Yes ☐	No ☑
Have you taken antacids, H2-receptor antagonists or acid pump inhibitors (drugs for ulcers, excess stomach acid, etc.) for periods of six months or more?	Yes ☐	No ☑
Are you hypersensitive to or do you react to any of the following in the environment: chemicals, detergents, dust, grass, mould, wormwood (*Artemisia*), perfume, pesticides, pollution, pollen, trees and plants or smoke?	Yes ☑	No ☐
Do you suffer from allergies or intolerances or are you hypersensitive to any foods (e.g. milk, wheat, peanuts) and/or additives (e.g. MSG, colourants, flavouring agents), which manifests as reactions in your digestive system or systemically (throughout your body)?	Yes ☐	No ☑

Do you suffer from chronic or persistent athlete's foot, ringworm, fungal infections in the groin, psoriasis or skin/ nail infections?	Yes ☐	No ☑
Do you suffer from frequent or chronic infections such as bladder infection, prostatitis, sinusitis or thrush?	Yes ☐	No ☑
Do you have cravings for sugar, sweets, desserts or similar?	Yes ☐	No ☑ ?
Do you have cravings for bread?	Yes ☑	No ☐
Do you have cravings for alcohol?	Yes ☐	No ☑
Score, Part 1:	*3*	*10*
Digestive system		
Do you suffer from diarrhoea or constipation?	Yes ☐	No ☑
Do you have problems with bloating, breaking wind or flatulence (frequent and foul-smelling wind)?	Yes ☑	No ☐
Do you often suffer from heartburn or reflux after eating?	Yes ☐	No ☑
Do you suffer from irritable colon or chronic inflammation of the intestines?	Yes ☐	No ☑
Do you have foul-smelling stools and/or mucous in your stool?	Yes ☑	No ☐
Do you suffer from haemorrhoids?	Yes ☑	No ☐
Do you suffer from frequent or recurring blisters/ulcers in your mouth?	Yes ☑	No ☐
Do you have bad breath and/or a (white) coating on your tongue?	Yes ☐	No ☑
Airways and mucous membranes		
Do you suffer from chronic colds (your nose is always running), chronically congested nose (especially when you wake up) and/or is your nose dry and/or itchy?	Yes ☑	No ☐
Do you suffer from a chronic cough (with phlegm) and/or breathing difficulties (wheezy breathing), lack of air and/or are you gasping for air?	Yes ☐	No ☑
Do you constantly need to urinate, do you urinate frequently and/or does your urine burn and/or is it cloudy?	Yes ☐	No ☑
Are your eyes always irritated or dry or your vision blurry, etc?	Yes ☑	No ☐
Do you constantly suffer from pressure in the ears, earache and/or fluid in your ears?	Yes ☐	No ☑

Muscles, joints, skin and other connective tissue		
Do you constantly suffer from aching muscles or do you feel weak?	Yes ☐	No ☑
Do you suffer from sore and/or swollen joints, especially when waking up in the morning?	Yes ☐	No ☑
Do you suffer from itching (including in vagina and anus), rashes, eczema or psoriasis?	Yes ☐	No ☑
Do you suffer from acne, especially on your upper body and/or on your face?	Yes ☑	No ☐
Central nervous system		
Do you frequently have mood swings, or become irritable or depressed?	Yes ☑	No ☐	sometimes
Do you have difficulty remembering, focusing or concentrating, do you feel confused or groggy and/or do you quickly become mentally tired?	Yes ☐	No ☑
Do you suffer from numbness, tingling, pins and needles and/or burning sensations in your extremities (hands, fingers, feet, toes, etc.)?	Yes ☑	No ☐	sometimes
Do you suffer from chronic headaches, a feeling of pressure in the skull, etc?	Yes ☐	No ☑
Do you feel dizzy or lightheaded or do you have problems with your balance or coordination?	Yes ☑	No ☐	sometimes
Metabolism and hormones		
Are you always feeling tired and exhausted, even if you get enough sleep?	Yes ☑	No ☐	sometimes
Do you suffer from low blood sugar (nervousness, fidgeting, dizziness) even if you eat regularly?	Yes ☐	No ☑
Do you often feel tired and sleepy during the day, especially after eating?	Yes ☑	No ☐
Do you have problems with water retention and oedemas (swellings) or do you feel bloated and heavy as the day wears on?	Yes ☐	No ☑
Do you have problems with your periods?	Yes ☐	No ☑
Do you have cysts in your breasts or ovaries and/or do you suffer from polycystic ovarian syndrome (PCOS)?	Yes ☐	No ☑
Immune defence		
Do you constantly suffer from aching muscles or do you feel weak?	Yes ☐	No ☑
Score, Part 2:	12	17

76

Part 1	Part 2	Interpretation
0–1 yes answers	0–13 yes answers	You probably don't have any problems with Candida or other "uninvited guests".
2–13 yes answers	14–29 yes answers	It's very likely that you have problems with "uninvited guests", e.g. Candida, parasites or bacteria that are harmful to your gastrointestinal tract and your health. You need to do something about it.

Sexy with healthy digestion

You need to fertilise your stomach garden. Your natural intestinal flora are as important for your intestines as natural fertiliser, earthworms and water are for your garden or your flowers. Natural lactic acid bacteria such as *Lactobacillus* and *Bifidus* strengthen the gastrointestinal part of your immune system. Buy them as food supplements. They are available from both chemists and health food shops. See more on www.pinetribe.com/thorbjorg/lactic-acid.

In addition to fibre, the following foods will help you maintain your own colony of normal digestive flora:

- Fermented dairy products like yoghurt, if you are able to tolerate milk – they should be plain, organic and completely without added sugar.
- Fermented vegetable juices: carrot juice, beetroot juice and other organic juices.
- Acidified or fermented vegetables, available from your health food shop – they normally consist of finely cut cabbage in glass jars (sauerkraut).
- Miso products made from fermented soy beans, brown rice or barley. Miso can also be purchased as a soup and is delicious.

Both putrefactive bacteria (which help us break down food, but cause problems if they get out of control) and fungi like *Candida albicans* can be controlled by eating antimicrobial food. There are ten times as many bacteria in your intestines as cells in your entire body. Your bacterial flora can weigh between 1 and 3 kg (about 2-6lb)! Digestive flora plays the starring role in the drama of your healthy immune system, and yet is completely overlooked.

Healthy mucous membranes

Even the most expensive cosmetic operation cannot fix an unhealthy internal mucous membrane. Create healthy mucous membranes in your gastrointestinal tract by living a calm, pure and considerate life in accordance with the lifestyle programme in this book. Avoid inflammation, oxidative stress (a chemical or biophysical stress in the body) and unwanted microorganisms. Otherwise, you will not be able to absorb the nutrients in food and food supplements.

You can throw out all unwanted guests, bacteria and fungi and/or parasites with my cleansing programme in weeks 5, 6 and 7.

Putrefactive bacteria help us break down and absorb undigested food, but they mustn't become too strong. That's what happens when proteins, or excess sugar or starch get stuck in your digestive system. If you also lack digestive enzymes in your stomach, your defence against foreign bacteria is weakened. They'll be able to travel through your gastrointestinal tract without being destroyed by the acid in your stomach, and will move into your intestines and cause problems.

Your feelings and your digestion

Your stomach talks to your brain via a phone line. This phone line is created by nerves that react to signals from both ends. The nervous system "sees", "listens" and "controls" your digestive tract from mouth to anus. I'm sure you know what I'm talking about. You feel your moods, fear, panic, worries and stress in your stomach either as a sinking feeling, agitation, pain or twinges, diarrhoea or constipation. Conversely, signals about a bad stomach, stomach ache, etc. are passed on to the brain, which then tries to balance and compensate. Clear speech and smooth communication from one end of your body to the other can be ensured using healthy, anti-ageing food from the recipe section of this book. This way, you can actually eat yourself into a better mood and get rid of depressive thoughts and melancholy.

The natural breakdown of proteins from e.g. meat, eggs and fish produces the amino acid tryptophan. The intestines use it to produce serotonin. Once the intestines have taken enough tryptophan to make the serotonin they need, the brain gets the rest. Serotonin is important for the entire central nervous system, the psyche and good quality sleep. If you have stomach problems, your intestines snatch all the tryptophan they can get to correct the damage to the gastrointestinal tract.

As a result, the brain lacks building material for the cerebral serotonin, and that's where the trouble starts. If you pay for therapy and counselling year after year to combat a depression that doesn't disappear, you may now understand why. The cause may be a bad stomach and not a life crisis. Consider whether you communicate with the wrong part of your body.

All's well that ends well...
The fact is that you should pass stools 1–3 times daily. It should be more or less odourless, well shaped, brown and preferably float.

Boosting your digestion – the best anti-ageing remedy

Your digestive system is the source of your youth. If your digestion works, you can get rid of used hormones and hormone-disturbing substances that age you and can make you very sick.

Your digestion is an amazing function. It also controls your mood and your sleep. There are therefore plenty of reasons to take good care of your digestive system. When I was a sugar junkie, I constantly suffered from stomach ache. I remember lying in a foetal position with unbearable stomach cramps. I would be bent over with stomach pain, embarrassed about my huge stomach, bloated like a soccer ball. People often made insulting comments about my "pregnant" stomach.

79

At that time, I was 18 years old and had almost never been kissed! I remember hours spent in vain on the toilet and chronic constipation.

I remember pimples and eczema on my face and hands and my extremely dry skin. I felt sorry for myself and was never really happy. My digestion played an important role in this regard. It took many years before I learned how to become healthy, happy and almost wrinkle-free.

Good digestion enables the proteins you eat to supply the necessary building materials for:

- Strong muscles that can carry you to the end of the world and stay flexible throughout your life without becoming stiff.
- Smooth and shiny mucous membranes to act as, for example, a barrier between your blood and intestines.
- Transport proteins that can move your hormones from one place to another and deliver messages about things like regular periods, ovulation, bone structure and good mood.
- Enzymes like digestive enzymes and detoxification enzymes.
- Healthy hair, skin and nails.
- Blood sugar balance and energy production.
- Antioxidants such as glutathione, that protect you against oxidative stress, poor liver detoxification and wrinkles.
- Control of and protection against inflammation that ages your body.
- A balance between a mental surplus of energy and prevention of depression, mental anxiety, fear, sleeplessness and stress.
- Your immune system, nervous system, hormone system, cardiovascular system and digestive system; a whole range of systems that are interdependent and whose proper function will be a major step towards reducing your biological age!

Good digestion enables the good fats you eat to supply the necessary building materials for:

- Cell membranes, transportation of nutrients to the cells and removal of waste materials from them so your skin is nourished from within and you avoid unnecessary wrinkles.
- Insulin sensitivity, proper burning of calories and good energy production.
- Hormones and good hormone production.
- Your brain and a well-functioning nervous system, producing joy and youthfulness.
- Mental stability and equilibrium, surplus energy, intelligence, logical thinking, concentration and memory.
- Your skin and its elasticity, flexibility and protection against sun, wind, pollution, untimely and unnecessary wrinkles and premature ageing.

Good digestion enables the good carbohydrates you eat to supply the necessary building materials for:

- Your digestion, which will be problem-free and regular if you get enough fibre.
- Balanced blood sugar.
- Energy production in the mitochondria, which benefits your entire body and mind.
- Detoxification of your liver so you can get rid of your used hormones.
- Your brain so it can think clearly.
- Your muscles so they can work properly and take you places! Several times a week!
- The creatures we keep in our intestines for our own benefit.
- Your good mood and trips to the movies!

Overgrowth of weeds in your stomach

If your digestion doesn't work, your garden will be overgrown with weeds and waste from your neighbours.

You'll suffer from:

- Bloating, wind, colicky pain, flatulence and bad breath.
- Breaking wind that stinks of rotten eggs or worse.
- Acid reflux, burning sensations in your stomach, gastritis or ulcers.
- Anal itching.
- Diarrhoea, constipation, explosive stools, a feeling of not being able to fully empty your bowel, distended stomach.
- Gurgling sounds from your stomach, bubbling and loud noises.
- Mucous or blood in your stools.
- Undigested food in your stools.
- Stinky stools: rotten eggs, sour, sweet or chemical smell.
- Pain: stomach ache, cramps, stabbing, shooting, deep, heavy, sharp, constant pains, regularly/after food/after certain types of food.
- Symptoms connected with food and eating: pain, wind, rashes, reactions in your airways, headaches, migraines, mental health symptoms and more.

If you have blood in your stools, you should see a doctor right away to check whether you suffer from a chronic intestinal disease.

The following symptoms can be a sign of infection in the intestines caused by bacteria, parasites and/or fungi. If the cause is the *Candida albicans* fungus (a form of yeast), it often affects both your intestines and your vagina. It can be a nasty affair with familiar symptoms:

- Pain and discomfort in your abdomen and vagina.
- Discharge that looks like cottage cheese and smells sour.
- Itching and stinging that can be unbearable.
- Pain and discomfort in connection with intercourse.

- Infections that flare up if you swim in a pool, in the cold sea, have intercourse, are stressed and, in particular, if you eat sugar, starch and grain products.

See what you can do to detoxify, in the antiage detox programme in Chapter 7.

Myth

We can only detoxify if we take a detox cure!

Fact

No, our bodies are designed to detox all the time, around the clock, every day of the week and throughout our lives. Proper detoxification is necessary for a youthful life and youthful looks that will be noticed by people around you. Proper digestion is an important part of the picture.

Feeling good without dysbiosis

Create harmony inside your body. Dysbiosis is an overgrowth of putrefactive bacteria and yeast fungi and/or uninvited guests: bacteria and parasites that colonise the intestines. They attract unnecessary attention from the immune system, gorge on the host's food, brew beer (yeast fungi) and in general have a party at the expense of the host. In addition, they often produce dangerous toxic and otherwise harmful waste products.

Consequences
- Infection causing topical damage.
- Leaky gut syndrome; creating holes in the stomach lining, which starts leaking.
- Diarrhoea or constipation or both in turn.
- Impaired digestion and poor absorption of nutrients.
- Impaired detoxification and accumulation of waste in the body.

Test yourself for dysbiosis – symptoms

- Your immune system reacts and works at top speed.
- Inflammation and oxidative stress.
- Tired immune system.
- So-called autoimmune diseases like rheumatism, chronic intestinal diseases, psoriasis, joint and muscle diseases.
- Neurological problems such as trembling, difficulty concentrating, memory loss, pins and needles.
- A weakened immune system and an increased risk of infection.
- Disturbed calorie absorption and use of nutrients.
- Skin problems: acne, pimples, sallow skin colour, lifeless skin, sagging skin and wrinkles.
- Allergies and food intolerance.
- Overloading of the liver and poor detoxification.

This is what my clients who suffer from accumulated toxins say about this condition

"I feel trapped in my own body and don't want to be in it."

"My muscles are always aching, and I have lost contact with parts of my body! It's as if it was dead."

"I had a shock when I saw a photo of myself among guests taken at a reception. My face was yellow and sallow-looking, and most of all I looked like a withered sunflower! It was a terrible sight, but good motivation for doing something about anti-ageing!"

This is how you get rid of toxins

- Minimise foreign toxic substances.
- Consume amino acids through your food.
- Boost your oxidative defence with vegetables, berries and antioxidants.
- Take micronutrients, especially the B12 and B9 methyl donors, but also B6.

- Get sulphur-containing amino acids from cabbage, onions, garlic and eggs.
- Eat phytochemical substances via the anti-ageing food in the recipe section of this book.
- Take a vitamin C supplement.
- Take bitter herbs like dandelion leaves, rocket and nettle.
- Strengthen your digestive system.
- Consider patching yourself with Y-AGE glutathione, carnosine and aeon from Life Wave. That will optimize your detox ability and short cut to the younger edition of your body. See www.pinetribe.com/thorbjorg/life-wave for more information.

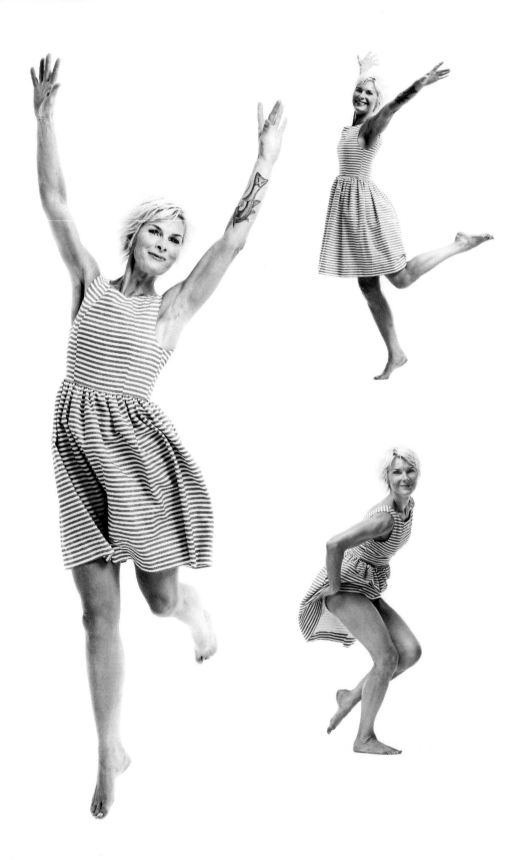

Exercise and become firm, young and energetic

Exercise keeps you young. Over-exertion makes you old. If you often train hard for two hours in a row, you'll get old before your time.

This week you're going to
- find your kind of exercise and get a healthy body through movement.

You'll need
- a beautiful, soft and practical tracksuit. If you're going to walk or run outside, you'll need the right clothing and good shoes from a specialty shop. Spend a day looking for the right clothing in sports or second-hand shops – or ask one of your girlfriends who has stopped training.

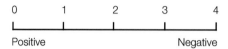

Positive   Negative

Each week you'll also need to write down what you have for breakfast, lunch and dinner every day. Don't forget to make a note of your snacks.

You can also see and fill out the table online at www.pinetribe.com/thorbjorg/my-charts

	Monday	Tuesday	Wednesday	Thursday	Friday	Saturday	Sunday
Energy 0–4 (describe)							
Digestion 0–4							
Bloating 0–4							
Weight							
Oedemas/swellings 0–4							
Headache 0–4							
Joint pain 0–4							
Muscle pains 0–4							
Bags/dark circles under your eyes/puffy eyelids 0–4							
Nose that runs/is congested 0–4							
Mucous in your airways 0–4							
Rash/eczema 0–4							
Dry skin 0–4							
Concentration 0–4							
Sugar cravings 0–4							
Mental state 0–4							
Feeling low 0–4							
Hormonal problems 0–4							
Irregular periods 0–4							
Hot flushes 0–4							
PMS 0–4							
PCOS 0–4							
Quality of sleep 0–4							
Exercise							

Avoid being bored to death doing Pilates or giving up your running programme for the umpteenth time. Your success with anti-ageing exercise depends on your exercise type. You'll find it below.

The "to go" type

Runs on adrenaline: quick fixes, energy in disguise – excitement, deadlines, café latte, lots of green tea, cigarettes, drugs. Generally the slim, fair type.

Problems and challenges

- Hyperactive
- Impatient
- Angry immune response such as eczema, asthma, hives
- Short-tempered
- Easily sunburned
- Food intolerances (often milk and gluten)
- Workaholic
- Sugar-dependent
- Not always sufficiently constructive

Strengths

- Normally slim (but not necessarily healthy)
- Quick to react
- Ambitious
- Eager beaver
- Hard-working
- Likes exercising
- Preferably fast aerobic training, masculine training, spinning, running, kickboxing, etc.

Recommended type of exercise

Needs to do lots of exercise, preferably spinning, running or fast swimming to burn off her energy. HOWEVER, should really dampen the adrenaline and stress response by doing yoga, Pilates, kayaking and meditation. Even if she doesn't think she has the patience to do it!

Food for exercise
- Needs protein at every meal
- Pure whey protein, tofu, fish, chicken, red meat
- Wholegrain products/seeds/nuts in the afternoon

Avoid
- Milk
- Cheese
- Wheat
- Raw tomatoes
- White potatoes
- Too many almonds and nuts (max. 10 at a time)
- Gluten is often a problem
- Sugar is almost a poison!

Dominant hormones

Glucagone, which empties the sugar deposits in the liver, and the stress hormones adrenaline and cortisol.

The "to stay" type

Androgynous. Boyish features. Plump to overweight, puts on weight easily, can have a hint of a dark moustache. Generally well balanced, but may experience internal turmoil because she doesn't know where to draw the line. Seeks tranquillity. Slow energy. Spends hours reading the paper. Perhaps a cup of hot chocolate with whipped cream or strong coffee with cream. Loves food, heavy food, even junk food, salt and chips.

Problems and challenges

- Slow metabolism
- Hormonal problems (PCOS, period problems, etc.)
- Constipated
- (Too) patient
- Heavy energy, tending to depressive
- Unwanted hair growth
- Can't be bothered with exercise
- Struggles losing weight
- Easily puts on weight around the stomach and waist
- Skinny legs
- Can't say no or does so awkwardly

Strengths

- Friendly
- Generally in tune with her masculine side
- Good at making decisions, not always the right ones though
- Dynamic
- Feet planted firmly on the ground

Recommended type of exercise

Nordic walking, brisk walking, swimming, yoga, Pilates, Thorbjörg's training programme.

1. 20 minutes – just me and my body.

2. 25–30 push-ups.

3. 100–200 sit-ups.

4. Training with elastic exercise bands. You can buy them at a sports store, or see **www.pinetribe.com/thorbjorg/elastic-band.**

   It is superb muscle training that you can do at home on the lounge floor, in your hotel room or even during a break at work.

5. Finish off with stretching and yoga/relaxation.

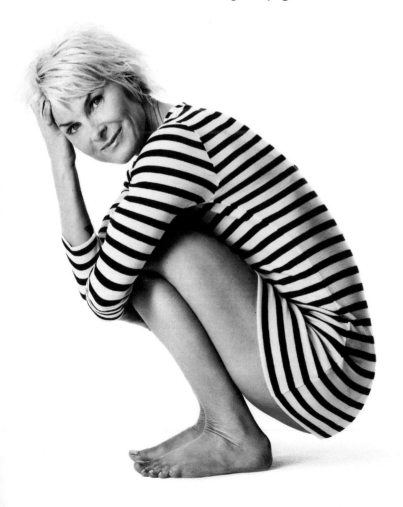

Food for exercise
- Eat regularly
- Proteins at every meal
- Wholegrain products only twice a day
- Eat rice protein powder

Avoid
- Soy products
- Raw vegetables, especially near relatives of cabbage such as broccoli and cauliflower
- Soy protein powder
- Alcohol

Dominant hormones
Thyroidea (thyroid gland) and testosterone.

The "yo-yo" type

This type is like someone on the edge of a war zone. The body is poised between fight and flight. This creates problems with to-ing and fro-ing, indecisiveness and anxiety. Wants to act and can't. Wants to rest, but can't relax. That's why I call it the yo-yo type – up and down.

Problems and challenges
- Overweight
- Puts on weight everywhere
- Can lose weight, but struggles to keep it off
- Tired
- Stressed
- Has a strong need for control, but loses it easily
- Tends to become depressed
- Mood swings, reacts to food, feelings, atmospheres
- Alternates between: happy and sad – hungry and full – focused and absent-minded – diarrhoea and constipation
- Not always in touch with herself

Strengths

- Warm
- Full-bodied
- Creative and very goal-oriented (once she's ready)
- Surplus energy once the decision is made

Recommended type of exercise

Only muscle-building exercises to begin with. Equipment at the gym. Yoga, Pilates, walking.

Food for exercise

- Protein with every meal
- Fish, a bit of tofu, but otherwise not much soy; whey protein and rice protein
- Fats with every meal (preferably omega-3 and butter)
- No grain products to start with, only quinoa and millet
- Stressed cavewoman in the 21st century – needs to be fed like a yo-yo: one week on a completely bread- and grain-free diet and one week on quinoa and millet and a slice of wholemeal rye bread or pumpernickel per day

Avoid

- Alcohol
- Potatoes
- Sugar is banned

Dominant hormones

Insulin and cortisol.

Now you know your type – these are your needs

Charac-teristics/ type	Type of exercise	Duration (minutes)	Week number	Supple-ment- before	Supple-ment - after
Hyper/ immune response "to go"	Spinning, running. Yoga, Pilates. Meditation or Thorbjörg's training programme.	45 60–90 15	2 3 Daily	Mg citrate, Lecithin granulate, Vitamin C, Green tea tab.	Q-10, Mg citrate
Andro-gynous/ metabo-lism/hypo "to stay"	Nordic walking, brisk walking. Yoga, Pilates. Thorbjörg's training programme.	30 60 15	3 2 Daily	Zinc, selenium, green tea tab, ome-ga-3	Mg citrate, Vitamin B
Metabolic/ war/ hyper/ hypo "yo-yo"	Muscle-building at the gym. Walks, Pilates. Yoga.	30 30 45	2 Daily 2	Co Q 10, R-ALA, Vitamin C, Mg, 2 gr L-Arginine	Mg citrate, Vitamin B

Key: Mg = Magnesium, R-ALA= Alpha Lipoic Acid, L-Arginine = amino acid.

95

Forget about pasta and protein bars – the following is your ultimate training nutrition.

- 400 ml water
- 100 ml unfiltered apple juice
- 2 tsp. spirulina powder.
  See www.pinetribe.com/thorbjorg/spirulina
- 1 tbsp. good quality fish oil or hemp oil
- 1 scoop whey protein or other protein powder
- 1 tbsp. beetroot crystals

For some this can be too heavy. In that case just mix the liquid with spirulina and beetroot crystals.

Mix well, and drink it with your training supplements 15-20 minutes before training. You can take the powder and the oil with you in a shaker and add the liquid just before training. Drink your morning shake afterwards, if you're training in the morning. Otherwise have your evening meal, which should also include root vegetables and a bit of rice or quinoa.

Exercise – why I can't live without it
- It's fun
- It's my alone time when I can unwind and empty my head of thoughts
- It makes me happy, especially when it's over
- It gives me confidence and self-esteem
- It's good for my mental health and improves my mood
- I sleep more soundly
- It improves my sex life
- My skin becomes more beautiful and supple (circulation)
- My pulse is perfect and my heart beats for love

- My partner loves it when I exercise because I become easier to get on with and more manageable (hmm!)
- I get extra energy for my everyday life
- My body becomes stronger
- My muscles become strong and healthy
- I'm happy with my weight
- Exercise and the food I eat maximise the insulin sensitivity in my cells
- I feel like a 20-year-old when spinning or running
- Yoga brings me closer to who I really am and want to be.

It should be enjoyable

If you're one of the many who haven't started exercising yet, then congratulations! You're lucky because you have a lot to look forward to! Go and find out what you enjoy: running, swimming, kayaking, cycling, circuit training? Indulge yourself with free trials in Pilates, yoga, body pump or dancing. Start today!

Sex is also a form of exercise

Sex releases emotions that promote a youthful body and mind. Training has the same effect. Exercise is training for the heart and the nervous system. Several studies show that running reduces stress symptoms. Regular sex also reduces negative stress. Exercise is therefore the new form of sex.

That doesn't mean that you should replace exercise between the sheets with a pair of running shoes. The two types of fun should complement each other. The physiological effect of orgasm is a release of endorphins. These are also released during running, but you have to run quite a long way and for a long time to produce the same amount of endorphins that you get from half an hour of sex with an orgasm. In addition, sex and running also produce nitrogen oxide, which stimulates circulation and the exchange of nutrients and waste materials in the cells. Intimacy, closeness, touch and light skin massage send beneficial messages to the nervous and hormonal systems.

Sex is the best anti-ageing medicine for both body and soul. If you don't get enough, you can do it yourself. Shop for sex toys, alone or with your partner. You can find decent, quality-conscious shops that stock adult toys that do not contain phthalates and other hormone-disturbing substances that you should avoid.

See www.pinetribe.com/thorbjorg/sex-toys.

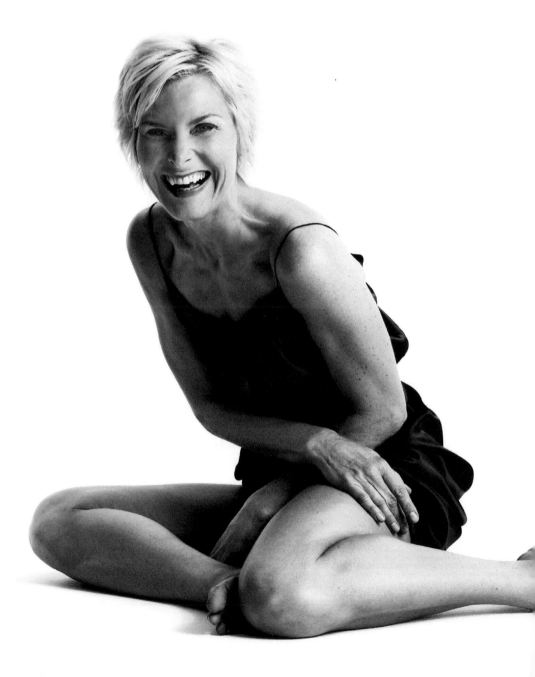

Anti-ageing detox programme

~~~~~~~

Detox and take a bite out of time

This week you're going to

- remove accumulated toxins and clear the way for future detoxification.

You'll need

- the products in the detox shopping list on page 103.
  You can also see and download the entire shopping list from
  www.pinetribe.com/thorbjorg/detox.
  Remember to keep the anti-ageing diary on the next page.

Once you start comparing food and health, it will become clear what makes a difference, what works and affects you, and what gives you negative symptoms or promotes good health. You become an expert on your own energy, body and psyche. This gives you power and responsibility.

It becomes easier to follow the programme if you get rid of negative expectations beforehand and don't feel sorry for yourself because you have to do without so much of the food you normally eat. Tackle the task with great expectations, curiosity and excitement and enjoy this new experience, even when the detox symptoms appear.

99

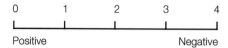

Positive   Negative

Each week you'll also need to write down what you have for breakfast, lunch and dinner every day. Don't forget to make a note of your snacks.

You can also see and fill out the table online at www.pinetribe.com/thorbjorg/my-charts

	Monday	Tuesday	Wednesday	Thursday	Friday	Saturday	Sunday
Energy 0–4 (describe)							
Digestion 0–4							
Bloating 0–4							
Weight							
Oedemas/swellings 0–4							
Headache 0–4							
Joint pain 0–4							
Muscle pains 0–4							
Bags/dark circles under your eyes/puffy eyelids 0–4							
Nose that runs/is congested 0–4							
Mucous in your airways 0–4							
Rash/eczema 0–4							
Dry skin 0–4							
Concentration 0–4							
Sugar cravings 0–4							
Mental state 0–4							
Feeling low 0–4							
Hormonal problems 0–4							
Irregular periods 0–4							
Hot flushes 0–4							
PMS 0–4							
PCOS 0–4							
Quality of sleep 0–4							
Exercise							

1. Cleansing
2. Elimination
3. Regeneration and improvement
4. Renewal and maintenance

1. Cleansing

Remove waste products, toxins, old used hormones, unwanted microorganisms in your intestines, excess acidity, additives and preservatives, colourants, antibiotics, medicine, solvents and chemical compounds, hormone-disturbing substances and everything else that prevents your body from shining with health and youthfulness.

You remove waste through your liver, intestines, kidneys, lungs and skin.

2. Elimination

Eliminate food that can cause "trouble" – all added sugar, gluten and all dairy products, and food that disturbs your immune system. Stress. If possible, excess use of mobile phones, television, computers, etc. Excess body fat. Excess bad cholesterol.

Bad connections and bad friends – you might as well remove them from your life while you're at it! Bad decisions. Bad and undesirable habits – smoking, alcohol, etc.

3. Regeneration and improvement

Good food and appropriate supplements to rebuild your intestinal flora, enzyme production, insulin sensitivity, mitochondrial function and energy, muscles, your liver's ability to detoxify, your hormonal balance, nervous system, sleep, mental energy, joy and balance, and so on.

4. Renewal and maintenance

A targeted anti-ageing diet; amino acids, fatty acids and supplements for cell renewal, gene expression, mucous membranes, energy, blood sugar balance, muscles, skin, neurotransmitter substances and hormones, the body's communication network, surplus energy, joy, confidence, self-esteem, control, sleep, circulation, blood pressure, body weight, etc.

Be prepared for the following when you detoxify

- Headache
- Constipation
- Diarrhoea
- Fatigue
- Bad breath
- Hunger pangs
- Irritation
- Itchy skin
- Anal itching
- Nausea
- Body odour/sweat
- Difficulty sleeping

Look forward to

- Better digestion and regular bowel movements.
- Fewer symptoms of chronic imbalance.
- Better concentration, focus and a clear head.
- Better mood and more joy.
- More energy and contentment.
- Fewer symptoms of food intolerance.
- Less accumulation of fluid in your body.

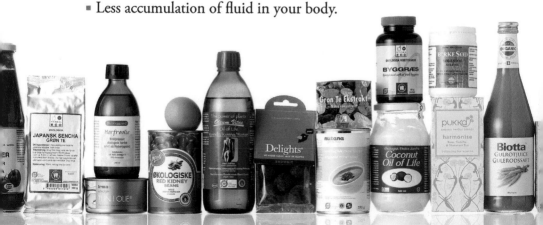

- More peace, harmony and balance.
- Less excess body weight.
- A smaller measurement around your waist and thighs.

Before you start

If you still drink coffee, now is the time to stop. Either go cold turkey or spend the rest of the week cutting down by one cup a day until you're coffee-free. Drink green tea instead of coffee. My favourite green tea is Original Green Tea Powder (see www.pinetribe.com/thorbjorg/green-tea).

Detox shopping list

You can see and download the entire shopping list at www.pinetribe.com/thorbjorg/detox.

Product	Dosage	Week used	Where to buy	Other
Fast And Be Clear	2 scoops morning (see detox shake recipe on p. 220)	5–7	Health food shops, see **www.pinetribe. com/thorbjorg/ fastclear** for more information	
Rice milk		5– 7	Most supermarkets and health food shops	
Cold-pressed extra virgin flaxseed oil	2 tbsp. in detox shake	All weeks	Most health food shops	
Lecithin granulate	1 tbsp. in detox shake	5–10	Most health food shops	Brain food
Ground cinnamon	1 tsp. in detox shake	5–7	All supermarkets	Insulin sensitivity and blood sugar
Lemons	Miscellaneous	All weeks	All supermarkets	Used in "detox shock", in water and cooking
Frozen berries	Miscellaneous	All weeks	Most supermarkets	In detox shakes and smoothies

Tofu	Miscellaneous	All weeks	In health food shops and well-stocked super-markets as well as Asian shops	In salads, soups and smoothies – see recipes
Chicken thigh or breast fillets		5, 7 and onwards	All supermarkets and similar shops	
Quinoa	100 g / 3 ½ oz	5, 7 and onwards	Most health food shops	NOTE! Choose one of the three grain types per day (quinoa, millet or brown rice) – see recipes
Millet	100 g / 3 ½ oz	5, 7 and onwards	Most health food shops	
Brown rice	100 g / 3 ½ oz	5, 7 and onwards	Most health food shops	
Detox herbal tea, liquorice root tea, Original Green Tea Powder	Drink as much as you like	All weeks, green tea max. 1–3 tea bags per day	Most health food shops. See **www.pinetribe.com/thorbjorg/herbal-tea** and **www.pinetribe.com/thorbjorg/green-tea**	NOTE! If you suffer from high blood pres-sure, only drink liquorice root tea in mode-ration
Cold-pressed extra virgin olive oil	Use in cooking and salads	All weeks		Use in food and as salad dressing
Cold-pressed extra virgin coconut oil	Use in detox morning shake and for frying	All weeks	Some supermar-kets and health food shops	Cooking and shakes
Epsom salts/ magnesium sulphate	As detox bath salts	Liquid detox in week 6	Most health food shops. See **www.pinetribe.com/thorbjorg/epsom**	Detox and cleansing
Miso soups	As you please	All weeks, but especially for "liquid days" in week 6	Most health food shops, some supermarkets and Asian shops. See **www.pinetribe.com/thorbjorg/miso**	For digestion and detox

Fruit from the basic shopping list in chapter 5: especially watermelon, pineapple and berries	Berries as you please, 1 slice watermelon and 1 slice pineapple at a time	All weeks and forever	Most health food shops and some supermarkets	
Vegetable stock/cubes	For soups, but in moderation due to the salt content	Especially during "liquid days" in week 6, but otherwise as you please	Most health food shops and super-markets	
Vegetable juice: carrot, beetroot, beetroot crystals, tomatoes, mixed	As you please	Especially during "liquid days" in week 6, but otherwise as you please	Most health food shops and some supermarkets. For the beetro-ot crystals see **www.pinetribe. com/thorbjorg/ beetroot**	Preferably organic brands or, even better, from freshly squeezed organic vege-tables
Pulses/chick-peas, mung beans or kidney beans (in tins or jars is fine)	As an ingredi-ent in salads, soups, etc.	From week 7	Most health food shops and some supermarkets	
Buckwheat cri-spbread, rice biscuits, qui-noa crispbread and other gluten-free crispbreads	Max. 2 at a time and max. twice daily (not in the morning)	From week 7	Most health food shops and some supermarkets. See **www.pinetribe. com/thorbjorg/ crispbread**	
Vegetables from the shopping list in chapter 5: especially broccoli, spi-nach, parsley, sweet pota-toes, carrots, rocket, lettuce, tinned toma-toes, beetroot, rosemary, basil and coriander	As much as you like and at least 600g (20 oz) daily and 300g (10 oz) broccoli three times weekly	All weeks and for the rest of your life!	Most supermar-kets and farmer's markets selling organic vege-tables	

Hemp glove or soft skin brush	Dry brushing of your skin	All weeks, but especially week 6	Some health food shops and chemists	
Yoga bands	Every day	All weeks	Health food shops and dance shops, various yoga places. See **www.pinetribe. com/thorbjorg/ elastic-band**	

Detox supplement list

You can see and download a list of the products and see suppliers for the whole list at **www.pinetribe.com/thorbjorg/supplements**.

Product	Dosage	From week	Where to buy	For how long	Other
Cold-pressed extra virgin flaxseed oil	2 tbsp.	Week 5 and for the rest of your life!	Most health food shops and some supermarkets	Always	
Cold-pressed extra virgin coconut oil	2–3 tbsp.	Week 5 at the latest, and for the rest of your life!	Health food shops and some super-markets	4–8 weeks	
Probiotics	1–2 capsu-les before breakfast and before bed	Weeks 5–10	Health food shops - or see my online supplement recom-mendations. **www. pinetribe.com/ thorbjorg/supple-ments**	All weeks and for a couple of months af-terwards	
Saccharomy-ces boulardii	1–2 capsu-les before breakfast and before bed	Weeks 5–10	Health food shops – or see my online supplement recom-mendations.	All weeks	

Tricycline®*	1 capsule three times daily	Week 5	Health food shops or see my online supplement recommendations.		After meals. Helps fight bacteria and fungi.
Milk thistle/St Mary's thistle/ Silimarin	2 capsules	Weeks 6–10	Health food shops or see my online supplement recommendations.		Liver and optimisation of glutathione, e.g. Siliverin from Solaray
Tricycline®*	2 capsules twice daily	Week 6			Smells of garlic for 10 minutes, after which the smell disappears. For new or old throat infections that can affect the immune response.
Tricycline®*	1 capsule three times daily	Weeks 7–8	See my online supplement recommendations.		
Vitamin B complex	1 tablet two to three times daily	Weeks 7–10	Health food shops – or see my online supplement recommendations.		Examples: NOW, Solgar B-100, Super B-Complex
Magnesium citrate	250 mg twice daily	Weeks 7–10	Health food shops - or see my online supplement recommendations.		
Vitamin C capsule / Lipo-spheric Vit C	1000 mg three times daily / 1 sachet a day	Weeks 7–10	Health food shops - or see my online supplement recommendations.		
Vitamin D3	2000 IU	Weeks 7–10	Health food shops - or see my online supplement recommendations.	All weeks	Should be taken all year round

CAUTION: Artemisinin is not indicated for pregnant or nursing women. Long-term administration (greater than 1 month) should be monitored by a healthcare practitioner and include liver enzymes and hemoglobin testing. Combining with antioxidants or iron may theoretically decrease effectiveness. Detoxification reactions may be experienced by some individuals. In rare cases may cause idiosyncratic liver dysfunction.

Vitamin E	350 IU	Weeks 7–10	Health food shops - or see my online supplement recom- mendations.		Must be mixed toco- pherols
Co-enzyme Q10	30 mg three times daily	Weeks 7–10	Health food shops - or see my online supplement recom- mendations.		Energy and mitochondria

Recipes for cleansing and detox

Refer to Chapter 13, the recipe section of this book and check out www.pinetribe.com/thorbjorg/recipes.

- Tofu salad
- Green smoothie
- Green soups with spinach and parsley
- Steamed fish with lemon and garlic
- Fried vegetables with prawns
- Bean salad with rosemary oil and garlic
- Smoothies
- Freshly squeezed or bought juice
- Fruit platter: pineapple, watermelon, berries
- Lemon water
- Boiled quinoa and tamari

Detox protein shake with Fast And Be Clear, (www.pinetribe.com/thorbjorg/fastclear). See recipe section in Chapter 13.

Week 5

You can eat the following
- Choose organic food – be inspired by the recipes in this book
- Protein shake – you need a good blender

Protein
- Fish, steamed, oven-baked or boiled
- Chicken
- Prawns
- Tofu
- Eggs

Vegetables
- Primarily broccoli
- Spinach
- Parsley
- Sweet potatoes
- Carrots
- Beetroot
- Zucchini (courgettes)
- Red onion
- Garlic
- Peeled and baked tomatoes
- Celery
- Spinach
- Rocket
- Romaine lettuce
- Fresh coriander
- Fresh basil
- Fresh rosemary

Grains

- Quinoa, whole or in flakes
- Millet, whole or in flakes
- Brown rice, whole, in flakes or as rice protein powder

Nuts and seeds

- Almonds, nuts, seeds

Herbal teas

- Green tea: Original Green Tea Powder
  (see www.pinetribe.com/thorbjorg/green-tea)
- Nettle
- Ginger
- Liquorice root
- Detox herbal tea

Fruit

- Lemon
- Watermelon
- Pineapple
- Berries: blueberries, strawberries and other berries – can be frozen
- Pomegranate and pomegranate juice without added sugar
- Aronia juice without added sugar

Spices

- Rosemary
- Fresh ginger
- Turmeric
- Cayenne pepper or chilli
- White or black pepper
- Sea or rock salt, unbleached

Avoid

- All bread
- Breakfast cereals with added sugar or honey
- Biscuits and cakes

- Sugar in any form
- Sweets and chocolate
- Dried fruit
- Potatoes
- White rice
- Dairy products (except pure organic butter)
- Red meat (beef, pork, lamb)
- Sliced meats (except pure organic chicken sausage)
- Bean sprouts (because of possible fungus spores)
- Coffee
- Alcohol
- Vinegar
- Yeast

Supplements in week 5

- Cold-pressed flaxseed oil
    - 2 tbsp. in your morning shake
- Cold-pressed extra virgin coconut oil
    - 2 tbsp. in your morning shake and/or for frying vegetables

Breakfast

- Detox shake – see the recipe section of this book
- Green tea
- Other herbal teas from the list above

Snacks

- Carrots or freshly squeezed / ready-made carrot juice without added sugar.
- Beetroot juice or beetroot crystals.
- Mixed vegetable juice: can be purchased ready-made.
- Green smoothie (see recipe section).
- Boiled brown rice or quinoa with additional cold-pressed extra virgin olive oil and a little tamari soy sauce.
- Berries, e.g. strawberries, blueberries or other defrosted berries.
- 1 slice of watermelon or fresh pineapple.
- Fresh pressed green juices.

Lunch

- Fried (in coconut oil) vegetables from the list above.
- Prawns, tofu or chicken (see the recipe section).
- Steamed vegetables from the list above.
- Steamed/baked fish or chicken (leftovers) or steamed tofu (see the recipe section).
- Salad of root vegetables, rocket, spinach and tofu or chicken (see the recipe section).
- Salad with celery, watermelon, pineapple, chives, coriander and prawns or tofu.

Evening meal

- Steamed fish, chicken or tofu.
- Baked fish, chicken or tofu.
- Boiled brown rice, quinoa or millet.
- Root vegetables, baked or steamed.
- Spinach, parsley, rocket and lots of steamed or lightly boiled broccoli.
- 2 tbsp. cold-pressed extra virgin olive oil.
- Lemon juice.
- Spices from the list above.

All day long

- Water with lemon or orange juice and zest.
- Green tea.
- Herbal teas from the list above.

Wellness, cleansing and everyday luxuries

Enjoy fresh air and go for a 30-minute walk every day. Gorge on fresh air with deep, healthy breathing. Breathe in and out consciously. Do yoga exercises on your lounge floor. Daily mindfulness. A quiet moment of reflection and meditation. Go for a swim every now and then.

Enjoy hot baths, spas, saunas or steam baths at your local swimming pool or spa bath. Enjoy a good laugh and positive thoughts, like "I am strong and beautiful" or "I accept my feelings and I love myself!" Read positive, self-development literature.

112

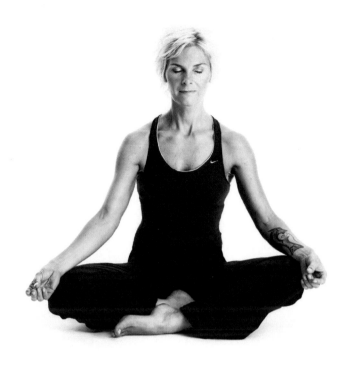

Cleansing through the skin

You need a soft skin brush, a hemp glove or oil and sea salt

1. Start by dry brushing your legs both front and back, from your ankles upwards.
2. Brush your buttocks with circular movements.
3. Brush the sides of your thighs.
4. Brush your stomach in a clock-wise direction.
5. Finally, brush both arms from your shoulders down.

Cleansing baths

Use Epsom salts (magnesium sulphate) in your bathtub: you need one cup for a full tub see www.pinetribe.com/thorbjorg/epsom. If you don't have a bathtub, take a footbath in a bowl and add ½ cup of salt. Afterwards, smear your body in healthy oils from chapter 11: *beauty: beautiful skin throughout your life.*

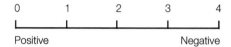

0   1   2   3   4

Positive   Negative

Each week you'll also need to write down what you have for breakfast, lunch and dinner every day. Don't forget to make a note of your snacks.

You can also see and fill out the table online at www.pinetribe.com/thorbjorg/my-charts

	Monday	Tuesday	Wednesday	Thursday	Friday	Saturday	Sunday
Energy 0–4 (describe)							
Digestion 0–4							
Bloating 0–4							
Weight							
Oedemas/swellings 0–4							
Headache 0–4							
Joint pain 0–4							
Muscle pains 0–4							
Bags/dark circles under your eyes/puffy eyelids 0–4							
Nose that runs/is congested 0–4							
Mucous in your airways 0–4							
Rash/eczema 0–4							
Dry skin 0–4							
Concentration 0–4							
Sugar cravings 0–4							
Mental state 0–4							
Feeling low 0–4							
Hormonal problems 0–4							
Irregular periods 0–4							
Hot flushes 0–4							
PMS 0–4							
PCOS 0–4							
Quality of sleep 0–4							
Exercise							

Week 6

You can eat the following

Days 1 and 2

Food plan as for week 5, but without chicken and eggs. Fish and tofu are still permitted during days 1 and 2 (and again on days 6 and 7).

Days 3, 4 and 5

An exciting liquid challenge. If you have a good juicer, use it now!

All solid food is forbidden, even tofu and nuts. Vegetables must be blended or boiled.

Begin day 3 with a "detox shock"

- 1 small glass lukewarm water (filtered)
- 4 tsp. Epsom salts
- 2 tbsp. cold-pressed extra virgin olive oil
- 2 tbsp. lemon juice

Mix the contents and drink everything at once. From the same glass, drink a glass of lemon water and then freshen your mouth with a couple of bites of orange or cucumber. Brush your teeth.

"Eat" the following the rest of the day

- Morning shake with cleansing Fast And Be Clear detox powder (see detox shopping list on page 103).
- Vegetable juice made from carrots, beetroot, wheat grass and barley – can be purchased ready-made.
- Green juice made from spinach, cucumbers, celery, lime and ginger.
- Beetroot crystals.
- Spirulina powder. See www.pinetribe.com/thorbjorg/spirulina

- Watermelon/strawberry soup/smoothie (see the recipe "Dreams on pink clouds").
- Green smoothie (see the recipe section - leave out dates, but use a little xylitol, if necessary).
- Green detox soups made from vegetable stock or organic vegetable stock cubes and plenty of fresh parsley and/or spinach (see recipe section).
- Vegetable soups, blended or clear (check ready-made soups in cartons or freshly made soups from your supermarket and see if they are "legal") – can be blended with a little tofu.
- Miso soups: rice miso, buckwheat miso and perhaps instant miso soup. Remember that the water shouldn't boil or the lactic acid bacteria in the miso won't survive. (See detox shopping list for where to buy.)
- Detox herbal tea or other good herbal teas.
- Green tea.
- Liquorice root tea or other herbal teas.
- Loads of water, with lemon or orange juice and zest if you want.

Days 6 and 7

- Repeat the food plan from days 1 and 2.

Supplements week 6

See www.pinetribe.com/thorbjorg/supplements for more information on suppliers near you.

- Cold-pressed extra virgin coconut oil in your shake, as before, 2–3 tbsp.
- Cold-pressed flaxseed oil in your shake, as before, 2 tbsp.
- Saccharomyces boulardii
    – 1–2 capsules after your daily "detox shock"
    – 1–2 capsules before bed.

- Probiotic
    - 1-2 capsules one hour after your "detox shock"
    - 1-2 capsules before bed.
- Tricycline®
- 1 capsule three times daily.

Congratulations! Fantastic! You're amazing!

You've come through what many people consider the most difficult and others the most amazing part of the cleansing programme! Fortunately, your cleansing will continue for another couple of weeks while you begin de-stressing and relaxing. At the same time, your body will get the peace and quiet it needs to repair and heal old damage and become ready for your anti-ageing food and nutrition.

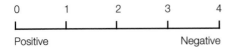

0   1   2   3   4

Positive   Negative

Each week you'll also need to write down what you have for breakfast, lunch and dinner every day. Don't forget to make a note of your snacks.

You can also see and fill out the table online at www.pinetribe.com/thorbjorg/my-charts

	Monday	Tuesday	Wednesday	Thursday	Friday	Saturday	Sunday
Energy 0–4 (describe)							
Digestion 0–4							
Bloating 0–4							
Weight							
Oedemas/swellings 0–4							
Headache 0–4							
Joint pain 0–4							
Muscle pains 0–4							
Bags/dark circles under your eyes/puffy eyelids 0–4							
Nose that runs/is congested 0–4							
Mucous in your airways 0–4							
Rash/eczema 0–4							
Dry skin 0–4							
Concentration 0–4							
Sugar cravings 0–4							
Mental state 0–4							
Feeling low 0–4							
Hormonal problems 0–4							
Irregular periods 0–4							
Hot flushes 0–4							
PMS 0–4							
PCOS 0–4							
Quality of sleep 0–4							
Exercise							

Week 7

You can eat the following

Food for the next two weeks

The same as for week 5, but once you finish week 7, you can begin to add:

- Buckwheat crispbread. See www.pinetribe.com/thorbjorg/crisp-bread
- Other sugar-free and gluten-free crispbreads.
- Rice biscuits.
- Pulses: chickpeas, kidney beans, mung beans and lentils – you can use preserved pulses in tins or jars, provided they're organic. If you get bloated after eating them, stop at once.

Supplements from now until the end of week 10
(see www.pinetribe.com/thorbjorg/supplements and the detox shopping list on page 103)

- Vitamin B complex 1 capsule twice daily
- Magnesium citrate 250–300 mg twice daily
- Vitamin C 1000 mg three times daily
- Vitamin D 2000-4000 IU daily
- Vitamin E as mixed tocopherols 250 IU daily
- Q10 100 mg once or twice daily

After week 10, continue with the supplements, but reduce vitamin C to 1000 mg daily.

Destructive thoughts prevent your body from collaborating with your deepest wishes and needs. Sabotage has never been the road to success.

Stop time by de-stressing and relaxing

~~~~~~

Find peace and quiet, and bring beauty and health back into your life

This week you're going to

- relax completely and understand why it makes you old if you don't take time out and allow yourself some peace and quiet every day.
- learn to change your own behaviour patterns and think positively.

You'll need

- a confined space.
- a sign saying "Do not disturb".

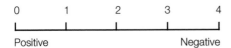

0   1   2   3   4

Positive   Negative

Each week you'll also need to write down what you have for breakfast, lunch and dinner every day. Don't forget to make a note of your snacks.

You can also see and fill out the table online at www.pinetribe.com/thorbjorg/my-charts

	Monday	Tuesday	Wednesday	Thursday	Friday	Saturday	Sunday
Energy 0–4 (describe)							
Digestion 0–4							
Bloating 0–4							
Weight							
Oedemas/swellings 0–4							
Headache 0–4							
Joint pain 0–4							
Muscle pains 0–4							
Bags/dark circles under your eyes/puffy eyelids 0–4							
Nose that runs/is congested 0–4							
Mucous in your airways 0–4							
Rash/eczema 0–4							
Dry skin 0–4							
Concentration 0–4							
Sugar cravings 0–4							
Mental state 0–4							
Feeling low 0–4							
Hormonal problems 0–4							
Irregular periods 0–4							
Hot flushes 0–4							
PMS 0–4							
PCOS 0–4							
Quality of sleep 0–4							
Exercise							

- Difficulty sleeping
- Chronic headache
- Fatigue and exhaustion
- Poor concentration and memory
- Muscle pains
- Excess weight or obesity
- Insufficient weight and undernourishment
- Inflammation, e.g. in joints and muscles
- Heart palpitations
- Sadness and weepiness
- Hopelessness
- Depression
- Lack of purpose
- Stomach aches and digestive problems

Case study

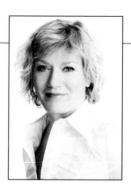

Gitte Barington

49 years old, self-employed.
Consultant, works in teaching,
consultancy and course development
within health and motivation.
Biological age: 41 years.

Before

When I was 40, I became seriously ill from stress and was unable to work for almost two years. I had a headache most days and often suffered from migraines immediately before my periods. Every month, I was completely hysterical and not myself for at least 24 hours. My muscles became stiff and when I got home from work, I sat for up to three hours on the couch, unable to do anything else.

When I resigned from my job, I didn't even have the energy to go and pick up the mail, and I slept for 15 hours a day. In addition to fatigue and a general lack of energy, my muscles were sore and my joints became more and more stiff. I woke up several times a night because my fingers were numb and aching, although I slept with splints on. It hurt to get up in the morning – my back was stiff and one wrong movement was enough for my back to lock up and give me pain for the rest of the day. In the morning, my feet also hurt when walking. I ended up being mildly depressed, as I never felt fresh, healthy and happy. I gained 10kg (about 20lb).

The turning point came during a discussion about retirement. I said I never wanted to be more than 55 years old. I didn't want to live any longer, as I could only imagine that my pains would get worse. Having three children and hearing myself saying this really woke me up, and I decided I had to keep trying different things until I found the solution to my physical problems. I decided I wanted to live a pain-free life and get my happiness and vitality back.

"When I resigned from my job, I didn't even have the energy to go and pick up the mail, and I slept for 15 hours a day. In addition to fatigue and a general lack of energy, my muscles were sore and my joints became more and more stiff."

Because of this I contacted Thorbjörg, who helped me change my diet. The first major thing that happened was that my skin became clear and beautiful for the first time in almost 25 years, which was fantastic. The next thing was that I recovered some of my energy, and the pain disappeared for periods at a time.

When I felt better, I unfortunately reverted to my old lifestyle and "forgot" how good I had felt. I once again had huge problems maintaining a consistent level of energy, and a medical check-up confirmed I had high blood pressure and a slightly elevated blood sugar level. That was a wake-up call. It was now or never. I couldn't postpone a healthy lifestyle any longer.

I contacted Thorbjörg again and went back to the lifestyle that makes me happy, gives me consistent energy and keeps me free from pain.

Now

I now have good, consistent energy throughout the day, provided that I remember to eat regular meals. I have beautiful, smooth and problem-free skin. I sleep soundly for eight hours every night without any pain in my fingers.

I wake up in the morning able to move my back, which no longer locks, and all my joints and muscles are pain-free, relaxed and supple. It no longer hurts to walk in the morning. My blood pressure and blood sugar are normal. My headaches are gone. I no longer suffer from PMS and no longer get hysterical or plagued by migraine attacks.

125

I am a new person. I'm happy, have plenty of surplus energy and mental resources, my self-confidence has soared and I now have the energy to exercise four times a week, which has turned my life around. I have a new body and a new life. I am grateful for that every day. Now I would love to live to older than 55, as long as I can remain pain-free, and my anti-ageing food and lifestyle ensure that. I have repeatedly tested whether it can really be true that food is so important. And it is. Every time I succumb to temptation and eat sugar or bread/gluten, my back pain immediately returns, I lose my energy and become grumpy and depressed. I lose my zest for life.

Read more great cases at www.pinetribe.com/thorbjorg/cases

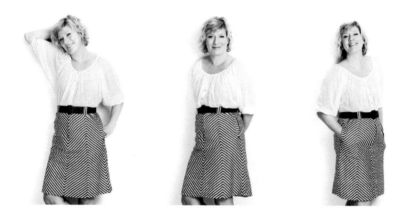

Days 1–4

Meditation and silence

Over time, a noisy lifestyle and stress make you old. The stress, noise and rush that often accompany working life, family life and social life can be too much for your nervous system and brain, which also need rest and cleansing.

What creates "noise" in your life?

- Plans and worries
- Shopping
- Dinner parties
- Having to buy birthday presents
- Mum's wedding anniversary
- Accounts
- Telephone conversations
- Work tasks that you have postponed
- Summer holidays, booking airfares
- The get-together with girlfriends next month (was it my turn?)
- Your kids' exams
- Your own exams
- Money worries
- Heartbreaks
- Weight problems
- Relationship problems
- Work problems

How to find rest

Few women manage to juggle their daily lives without confusion, stress and dark circles under their eyes. You need to close your door, sit down and daydream for five minutes. Make it part of your daily anti-ageing routine.

This is what you do

Invent your own favourite place, perhaps a beach, a mountain top with a fantastic view or a place in the jungle with beautiful sounds and moist heat on your cheeks.

Sit there for five minutes and empty your head. It takes practice because your conscious mind constantly tries to interfere, with new plans and worries. Gently push them out of your mind and return to your special place. You can do this no matter what kind of job you have, or wherever you are. If you're in your own office, where people come and go, put a sign on the door saying: "Noise-free zone. Do not disturb!"

You make contact with the alpha waves in your brain.

Why is that so important? Because it affects the hormones that cause natural ageing. The growth hormone HGH, which is produced in the brain, only becomes active when we enter the deep stage of sleep called NREM (non-rapid eye movement) sleep. That's where the alpha waves are activated, and this happens during meditation. People who do yoga and meditate regularly are calmer and have more surplus energy. I'm sure they're also more friendly and tolerant, towards others and themselves. This especially benefits the "to go" type described in the exercise test in this book. You need something to balance your masculine lifestyle of stress, speed, extroversion and strenuous sport.

I remember a lovely young girl who once came to see me. She was a basketball player, big, muscular, a bit overweight, an achiever and sugar-dependent. A typical adrenalin-fed type. I put her on an anti-ageing diet, and together we got her sugar dependency under control. That was really good for her weight and many sports injuries. However, she wasn't really in touch with herself, her feelings, who she was and what she really wanted – apart from being the best on the team. She needed something to counter all that masculinity.

There was too much earthiness, so to speak, and no air or water. I suggested she should do meditation and yoga and find out how she could introduce a bit more laughter in her daily life. She did. I met her two months later, and the difference was striking. She was more beautiful, softer, more attentive and warm. She had become hooked on meditation and loved her yoga lessons because she could clearly feel that, while becoming more supple physically, this "brain sport" brought her into contact with other, more gentle and sensitive sides of herself that she wasn't aware of. "I had no idea that I had all these feelings! I'm getting softer and everybody notices and asks me what I'm doing. Now I no longer have to be the best on the team, as long as I'm part of the best team," she says.

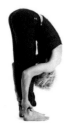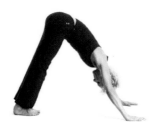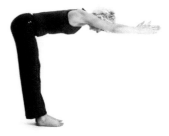

Day 5

Smile at the world

If you want more joy in your daily life, smile at the people you meet in the street, the woman sitting beside you on the bus or standing next to you in the queue at the airport, the waiter who brings your food, your colleagues or your employer. There's a great chance they'll smile back.

Day 6

Rejuvenating thoughts

Destructive thoughts prevent your body from collaborating with your deepest wishes and needs. Sabotage has never been the road to success. Rejuvenating thoughts help you make your wishes come true and promote joy, energy, surplus mental energy, good diet, beauty and health.

It makes you younger to have a meaningful job and good contact with yourself, your friends and family. If your approach to life is that your happiness and success depend on your husband or sweetheart, your children, the love and acceptance of others or on the time being just right, your needs might never be fulfilled.

When is it the right time to stop eating sugar or smoking, and to start eating rejuvenating, sexy morning shakes and taking exercise?

What prevents you from doing it right now? Do you recognise that inner voice that sabotages your good intentions by saying:

- "No, it's much too hard to give up sugar, and I can't be sure it'll help."
- "It takes too much time to prepare all that healthy food, and I'll probably have to shop in ten different places."
- "Being healthy is very expensive."
- "I don't know how to do it."
- "I can't cook."
- "I'm fat and ugly, and it's not going to change."
- "I'll start next Monday!"

and other negative barriers along the same lines? Words are like food. They contain information that either releases and liberates, creating possibilities and development, or locks you into unhealthy patterns that you can't escape from. Your body, your nervous system and your hormones also react to words from your brain. You can choose the type of communication that sabotages and limits you, and stresses and ages your body, or you can choose a constructive smooth communication that keeps you young.

Why is negative communication with yourself so bad for you?
- You get tired.
- All the tension weighs you down.
- Your moods fluctuate.
- You become sad.
- You develop muscle pain.
- You suffer from headaches.
- You sleep poorly.
- You become irritable.
- It destroys your self-esteem.
- You become frustrated.
- You feel you're not good enough.
- You are stressed.

130

- You get stomach aches.
- You get stuck in bad energy.

How to break your negative pattern.

- Get out of your comfort zone.
- Challenge yourself.
- Go out at night and look men in the eyes.
- Say to yourself: here I am, and this is what I look like.
- Don't look away when you catch a man's eye.
- Take time out for yourself (six minutes per day will do) for positive self-talk.
- Positive thoughts: I can do everything, I'm beautiful, living healthily is easy, I put myself first, I love spending money on my health. Invent more.
- Buy an imaginary pair of scissors and cut up all negative thoughts as soon as they pop up.
- Buy a vibrator.
- Think of yourself as strong, youthful, healthy and sexy. It works!
- Behave as a strong, youthful, healthy and sexy woman. That also works!
- Buy dark chocolate next time.
- Book a trial session at your fitness centre.
- Go to a male strip show (this is a really good exercise in getting outside your comfort zone).

Day 7

Clarification

Who are you, where are you going, how?

We all ask ourselves these questions from time to time, and now that you have decided to do something about your diet and lifestyle, you may need help to clarify and achieve your goals. I both like, and am inspired by Debbie Ford, www.debbieford.com.

It's not the stress itself that determines whether it harms us and makes us old before our time. It's the way we handle the stress that's all-important, and the amount of stress you expose your body to throughout your life in the form of toxins, poor quality food, too much sugar and not enough exercise. We're all very different, including in the way we handle stress. Our ability to handle stress is influenced by

- Surplus mental energy
- Maturity
- Life experience and baggage
- What we eat
- Anti-oxidative stress
- Sleep and quality of sleep
- Exercise

MEDICAL		
Have you ever been diagnosed with clinical depression that has lasted more than six months?	Yes ☐	No ☑
Do you have trouble falling asleep and/or do you wake up too early?	Yes ☐	No ☑
Do you suffer from chronic inflammation (asthma, arthritis, migraines, etc.)?	Yes ☐	No ☑
Do you suffer from an autoimmune disease (osteoarthritis, Crohn's disease, lupus, etc.)?	Yes ☐	No ☑
Do you suffer from any allergies all year round?	Yes ☑	No ☐
Have you been diagnosed as an adult with hypothyroidism or any other problems with your thyroid gland?	Yes ☐	No ☑
Do you have high cholesterol, high blood pressure and/or high blood sugar?	Yes ☐	No ☑
FEELINGS		
Do you feel worried or overwhelmed, or do you easily become frustrated about the things you're responsible for in your daily life?	Yes ☐	No ☐

Do you experience psychological or emotional conflict in your interactions with your husband/partner, your relatives, friends or colleagues on an almost daily basis?	Yes ☐	No ☑
Are you worried or afraid for a lot of the day?	Yes ☐	No ☑

PHYSICAL

Do you suffer from poor digestion, constipation, infrequent bowel movements (less than once per day), acid reflux and/or stomach ulcer?	Yes ☐	No ☐
Have you gradually but consistently gained weight as you have grown older and/or do you struggle to achieve permanent weight loss?	Yes ☐	No ☑
Are you constantly tired and/or does your energy level drop as the day goes on?	Yes ☐	No ☑
Do you exercise less than 30 minutes at a time, less than three times a week?	Yes ☐	No ☑
Do you often catch colds or flu, or get cold sores, especially after prolonged periods of stress, and does it take you longer than normal to recover?	Yes ☐	No ☑
Do you suffer from chronic/repeated infections?	Yes ☐	No ☑
Do you have wounds that are slow to heal?	Yes ☐	No ☑
As an adult, do you suffer from acne or greasy skin, especially on your upper body?	Yes ☑	No ☐
Do you experience that you become allergic/intolerant to more and more foods and/or that you have started becoming hypersensitive to things like chemicals, additives in your food, perfume, detergents, solvents or similar?	Yes ☐	No ☑
Do you suffer from headaches at least once a week?	Yes ☐	No ☑

SOCIAL

Are you always busy and/or running late?	Yes ☐	No ☑
Do you find it hard to say no and often end up taking on too much?	Yes ☑	No ☐

NUTRITION

Do you feel unwell almost daily after eating fat, salt and/or sweet food and junk food?	Yes ☐	No ☑
Do you drink more than one standard unit of alcohol or ½ litre of caffeinated drinks (coffee, coke, black tea, etc.) per day?	Yes ☑	No ☐
Do you skip meals, allow yourself less than 20 minutes to eat meals and/or fail to eat at more or less regular times every day?	Yes ☐	No ☑

Count the number of yes answers. Each "yes" represents circumstances, events or conditions that cause your body to increase its production of the stress hormone cortisol. The more times you answered yes, the greater the risk that your adrenal glands are producing cortisol continuously, that is, that your body thinks every day is an emergency situation. That ages you.

NUMBER OF "YES" ANSWERS	YOUR CORTISOL STATUS
1–6	Your cortisol levels may be too high.
7–12	Your cortisol levels are probably too high.
13–25	You have very high stress and cortisol levels and an increased risk of early ageing. You risk having to struggle with the illnesses that come with premature ageing. If you're already sick, there's a great risk your condition will worsen.

What makes you old before your time?

Cortisol is a stress hormone that is useful in potentially dangerous situations. When a person needs to give a fight or flight response, the body produces cortisol and adrenalin. Cortisol sends a message about the emergency situation and encourages the body to save its strength. The body turns off the maintenance of muscle mass, regeneration, bone mass and energy production. This is an advantage in critical situations, but a disadvantage if this emergency situation becomes the body's everyday experience. It causes the body to slowly decay. That's why you have to avoid long-term stress that can cause problems like:

- Reduced resistance to infections.
- Loss of bone mass.
- Insulin resistance and blood sugar problems.
- Loss of muscle mass.

- Increase in fatty tissue.
- Your brain centres shrink, including the hypothalamus and the hippocampus, which is where your feelings are located.
- Reduced energy production.
- Depression and altered brain chemistry.
- Slow healing of wounds.
- Oedemas / swellings.
- Changes in your digestive function and the flora in your gastro-intestinal tract.
- Difficulty sleeping and altered sleep patterns.
- High cholesterol, triglycerides and blood pressure.

Let the salmon teach you how to live a long life

The Canadian salmon can teach you a few things about how excessive production of stress hormones can make you old before your time. The male salmon swims through the Atlantic and Pacific Oceans on its way to the large rivers in Canada. It must fertilise the eggs laid by the female salmon to make salmon babies. It's a long, long swim.

Driven by instinct and a built-in genetic compass, it swims thousands of miles. As it approaches the coast of Canada, the current becomes stronger, and towards the end of its journey, it has to fight the current and literally jump up rivers and waterfalls. This requires enormous strength and the salmon must therefore produce huge amounts of the stress hormone cortisol. Once it has completed its mission and spread its sperm over the eggs, it dies of old age, as a result of stress. The enormous effort and excessive production of stress hormones messes up its hormones. Daddy salmon dies of old age although he isn't physiologically old.

What can we learn from this? We can learn that the same could happen to us. Stress can cause hormonal problems, which can disturb the natural ageing process and add years to our age. Stress can cause wear and tear on our cells so our body becomes weak, floppy, grey and old. Stress can be caused by many different factors both inside and outside the body. Women don't necessarily all respond to stress factors in the same way.

Stress can be caused by heartache, lifestyle, unhealthy food and much more. The body reacts in the same way whether the cause is internal or external, often with premature ageing as a result, and fatal consequences.

External factors that cause you to age from stress

This is called exogenous stress. It's stress caused by factors outside our bodies that affect our entire organism.

Examples
- Divorce
- Loss of a friend, spouse or family member
- Change of residence
- Wedding
- Pollution, smoke, noise and smells
- Too much work
- Poor working conditions
- Heartache
- Financial problems
- Unfinished projects

We can influence some of these stress factors, such as change of residence. Others are difficult to change, e.g. smell and pollution.

Internal factors that cause you to age

This is called endogenous stress. It's the result of factors that occur within our bodies and affect us.

Examples

- Blood sugar imbalance
- The immune system's response to food we can't tolerate – allergies and food intolerances
- Lack of good nutrients
- Lack of vitamins, minerals and trace elements
- Poor ability to detoxify, e.g. in the liver
- Inflammation
- Oxidative stress
- Accumulation of toxins
- Foreign or undesirable bacteria, fungi or viruses in the intestines or elsewhere in the body

This is what happens inside you when you get stressed

What happens in your body when you're stressed takes place in several stages. Whether you get through them all unharmed depends on whether you have sufficient nutrients, strength and healthy food stockpiled in order to resist the pressure from a stressful lifestyle or stressful food and thoughts.

Stage 1 – alarm

When your body is exposed to stress, for example in connection with low blood sugar (internal stress), your body reacts by becoming alarmed and producing stress hormones. You may feel unwell, dizzy or tired and go to bed. Or you might become ill because it was too much of a downer for your body.

That's what Hans Selye calls the "alarm phase" in his famous stress model, first described in his book *The Stress of Life*, for which he was nominated for the Nobel Prize.

Stage 2 – adaptation

Selye calls the next stage the "adaptation phase". When the body is exposed to repeated stress such as low blood sugar, poor health and fatigue, the result is a domino effect with systems such as high blood pressure, excess weight and inflammation. The body tries to adapt to the circumstances. The organism and the adrenal glands can only do so if they're sufficiently protected with the right food, including vitamin C, pantothenic acid (B5) and lecithin.

In fact, a certain amount of stress is necessary for an organ to work optimally. Stress only ages you if it's a frequent visitor in your body, for instance if you work too much or eat unhealthily all the time– and if your body cannot resist because it lacks nutrients and mental strength. You experience harmful stress as fatigue and low spirits most of the time. You might even forget what it's like NOT to be tired and off colour. You might begin to think that all normal busy people feel like that, until you get sick, sleep poorly, get pains in your joints and muscles, have constant headaches, gain weight and/or lose muscle mass and struggle getting through the day.

Stage 3 – exhaustion

Eventually, you reach the stage of exhaustion. Your biochemistry plays up and your hormonal system goes into shock along with the rest of your body. It's a total meltdown, and it ages you. Once you reach this stage, you quickly become 10–20 years older than your biological age. The stress load is identical to the one the salmon experiences after swimming thousands of miles against the current. The salmon dies from it, so this is a serious matter. Your immune system and your body have tried in vain to grab your attention with fatigue, illness and other clear messages. You continued, perhaps because you could no longer hear the alarm bells or had forgotten what they sound like.

Selye's stress model can be used to explain negative symptoms and declining health. You can use it to see patterns in your life that have to be changed for you to get better. The problem could be your working life, what you eat, how you sleep or many other things. Let me give you an example. If you continue eating food that you actually can't tolerate, like for example dairy products and sugar, your body will be under constant stress, and this will cause problems. It causes oxidative stress and inflammation in your body, which weakens you and makes you sick and old. Another example could be that you have a job you don't like – one that doesn't give you the challenges you need or enough money in your pocket. It stresses you and becomes the start of the domino effect.

Self-help against stress

If you stress your body with a life, food or actions that go against your nature, your adrenal glands produce the stress hormones adrenalin and cortisol. Your adrenal glands need vitamin C, vitamin B5, lecithin, exercise, love and good sleep. This enables them to resist pressure over a period of time.

Thorbjörg's survival guide for stressed women

This is how to tackle stress and avoid becoming old and ugly.

Take supplements (also see the detox shopping guide on page 103 or www.pinetribe.com/thorbjorg/detox)

- Vitamin C, 1000 mg, morning, noon and night before going to bed. Eat berries, oranges and red bell peppers when you're stressed.
- Fish oil, 3–10 g per day when you need to recover.
- Vitamin B5 (pantothenic acid), 200 mg before bed. Eat avocados, tuna and chicken.
- Lecithin granulate in your morning drink. See the recipe for "Sexy morning smoothie" in the recipe section of this book. Add 1 tbsp. Take another 1 tbsp. before bed in a bit of soy milk. Have it with a banana.
- If you already take vitamins C and B as described in chapters 5–7, you should take max. 1000 mg more. Remember to cut down slowly over the next two weeks if you have been taking more than 2000 mg vitamin C for an extended period of time (three weeks or more). Consider taking Ashwagandha (Indian Ginseng). This herb is really helpful for adrenal stress.

De-stressing behaviour

- Make sure you sleep soundly for seven to eight hours every night. Go to bed early. Consider using Silent Night patch from Life Wave. See www.pinetribe.com/thorbjorg/life-wave
- Exercise four or five times per week.
- Get your daily hug and be open to love.
- Feel your vulnerability and accept it. It can teach you a lot.
- Get help from a good coach.
- Eat the food described in this book.

De-stressing food

Broccoli that grows in an unsprayed field, exposed to sunlight, unprotected against attacks by beetles and other insects that want to eat it, is exposed to stress. You can use that to your advantage. The broccoli has mobilised its own immune defence. This immune defence is the production of substances called secondary substances or phytochemicals. When you eat broccoli, you can take advantage of this defence system for free. That's why I love food full of phytochemicals. They strengthen my defence against harmful and ageing free radicals. The dark, preferably purplish-green broccoli is particularly good. These colours show that the broccoli is stressed and full of the good substances we want to consume.

Fruit, berries and other dark green vegetables have the same protective and de-stressing properties.

Boost your genes and cells

Why make do with what your parents gave you?

This week you're going to

- optimise your cells and marvel at how much you can influence your genes and thereby your ageing process.
- throw out the worst nasties that steal your youth.

You'll need

- a shopping bag and purse. You're going shopping for power food supplements, if you haven't done so already.

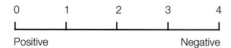

Each week you'll also need to write down what you have for breakfast, lunch and dinner every day. Don't forget to make a note of your snacks.

You can also see and fill out the table online at www.pinetribe.com/thorbjorg/my-charts

	Monday	Tuesday	Wednesday	Thursday	Friday	Saturday	Sunday
Energy 0–4 (describe)							
Digestion 0–4							
Bloating 0–4							
Weight							
Oedemas/swellings 0–4							
Headache 0–4							
Joint pain 0–4							
Muscle pains 0–4							
Bags/dark circles under your eyes/puffy eyelids 0–4							
Nose that runs/is congested 0–4							
Mucous in your airways 0–4							
Rash/eczema 0–4							
Dry skin 0–4							
Concentration 0–4							
Sugar cravings 0–4							
Mental state 0–4							
Feeling low 0–4							
Hormonal problems 0–4							
Irregular periods 0–4							
Hot flushes 0–4							
PMS 0–4							
PCOS 0–4							
Quality of sleep 0–4							
Exercise							

Day 1

Introduce vitamins and minerals

If you are short of vitamins, minerals and trace elements because you've been eating modern food lacking in nutrition, you disturb your genes' repair system. Your internal inspector becomes under-nourished and tired, and this affects her commitment and work. She becomes slack and doesn't discover errors and damage in your genes. She might not be in time to prevent damaged genes from being copied millions of times in your body. A sufficient number of errors will have catastrophic consequences for your inspector's work.

- Cancer
- Premature biological ageing
- Reduced/weakened mitochondrial function (energy production in your cells)
- Cardiovascular diseases

Vitamins and minerals – an anti-ageing wonder cure

In Hollywood, the superstars get their "vitamin shots" like it's the most natural thing in the world. It's obvious that high doses of vitamins and minerals work 100 times better than creams and serums. Unfortunately, not everybody can get vitamin injections. I therefore thank God for the Internet, which enables me to look after my beauty by getting much higher doses than those recommended on the labels of standard multivitamin products. I choose to go by Optimum Daily Allowance (ODA) to optimise my body's natural function instead of Recommended Daily Allowance (RDA). For many years, I have followed the recommendations of American researchers regarding high doses of vitamins and minerals – the recommendations of people like Bruce Ames instead of mainstream European advice. My health, skin, body and general condition are evidence that it works. My way of saying it is: normal Western food doesn't deliver the goods and neither does a standard vitamin tablet.

143

Research into energy and ageing is relevant for all anti-ageing women...and men! Do you get micronutrients in your food? Do you want to make do with the small doses of vitamins, minerals and trace elements that are recommended by the health authorities? In my view, the recommended dosage is not sufficient to protect us against the challenges inflicted upon us and our genes by a typical Western lifestyle.

Bruce Ames is a biochemistry professor and researcher. He is renowned for his research into genes and ageing. One of his conclusions is that a lack of micronutrients increases the rate of damage to our genes. Lacking these micronutrients can make you sick and old before your time. Without them, your body can't gather important information from your genes. It means that your body misses out on the instructions it needs for looking good and being healthy and strong. Neither can it get told to minimise wrinkles, and fight chronic intestinal and cardiovascular diseases, and so on.

If you skipped chapters 5–7 and haven't already been out shopping for vitamins, the supplements you should be taking daily are described below.

- Vitamin B complex – 1 tablet twice daily
- Magnesium citrate – 250–300 mg twice daily
- Vitamin C – 1000 mg three times daily during program
- Vitamin D – 2000-4000 IU daily
- Vitamin E as mixed tocopherols – 250 IU daily
- Q10 – 100 mg twice daily

You can buy these products at your local health food shop or see www.pinetribe.com/thorbjorg/supplements.

Days 2–3

Hurray – you can influence your genes

There's no doubt that your genes contain very important information, but 65% of their behaviour can be attributed to the environment and your lifestyle – these determine whether your unfortunate genes are able to express this information. Hello! That's a bit of a wake-up call, isn't it? It means that you have the responsibility, power and endless opportunity to influence anything from your age and looks to your health. You can now act in a meaningful, conscious, creative and loving way to make the best of the body you have. Anti-ageing food is a very important part of the options that you have. Exercise, love and positive thoughts are other components. There's a connection between your genes and your environment. Our genes are not entirely responsible for how well we are or become, or whether we develop diseases – or for how we age or keep fit.

You determine whether you want your genes to express beauty and health or the opposite. Eat whole, genuine food that contains all the right information for your body. Take basic vitamins, minerals and antioxidants daily. Be positive and active, both physically and mentally.

Eat

- Leafy green vegetables, beetroot and good quality meat.
- The basic supplements recommended in this book.
- Alpha-lipoic acid and acetyl-L-carnitine – anti-ageing supplements that work! You can buy them in your local health food store or supermarket, or see www.pinetribe.com/thorbjorg/lipoic-acid

You deserve to get 100% of the micronutrients that you need. They will keep you young and strong throughout your life.

It's not only your internal gene inspector that's dependent on micronutrients. The telomerase enzyme – the main actor in the drama of life, death and age – also needs vitamins and minerals to do its anti-ageing job properly.

Day 4

How long would you like to live? Boost your genes!

The size of your telomeres determines how long you're going to live. Dr Konrad Hayflick, researcher in ageing, says so. So what are telomeres?

Your chromosomes are held together by strings. These strings are called telomeres. They are like sticks that support orchids and keep them straight and upright. If you remove the stick, the flower collapses, is destroyed and dies. With age, telomeres become shorter and shorter until they disappear. They become shorter and disappear because of cell division, and you can do something about that. Some of the things that cause frequent cell divisions are inflammation and oxidative stress in your body.

If you live the anti-ageing lifestyle and follow my advice for the rest of your life, you'll reduce oxidative stress and inflammation in your body. Inflammation is caused by too much sugar, white bread and grain, or other food resulting in a high glycaemic load.

Good news – telomeres can be both repaired and reconstructed

You use the telomerase enzyme to repair the strings that will keep you alive for many years to come. This enzyme is dependent on the presence of some very special methylating micronutrients. You can do your bit to help repair your telomeres by taking the following vitamins and food supplements.

146

- Vitamins B12, B9 and B6 in the form of vitamin B complex.
- Betaine and choline, which are contained in vitamin B complex, from my online recommendations page at www.pinetribe.com/thorbjorg/betaine, as well as leafy green vegetables, beetroot, beetroot juice and beetroot crystals (see www.pinetribe.com/thorbjorg/beetroot-crystals)
- Astragalus (astragalosides)
- Omega-3 fatty acids

If you already take vitamins as described above in day 1 of this chapter, don't take any more.

Days 5–7

Eat food packed with nutrients

When you provide your body with nutrients, it looks after your most important organs first: your heart, kidneys, liver and brain. What's left is used for the rest of your body: your skin, immune defence, and your hormonal and nervous systems.

If you have dry or wrinkled skin, you can be quite sure that you're lacking in healthy fats. Your body has distributed fat to the vital internal organs, but there wasn't enough to also nourish your skin. If you have frequent infections, this can also be due to an undernourished immune system – just as trouble with your periods and menstrual cycle can be caused by a lack of good fats. Depression can be the result if you have insufficient protein in your food to support your nervous system.

That's why it's vital to eat proper, unprocessed food without chemicals, but packed with quality vitamins, minerals, trace elements and antioxidants. Natural, organic and unrefined foods speak a language your genes understand. And when your food communicates nicely with your genes, they'll express themselves properly and healthily so you can begin feeling that you're actually living and not just surviving.

Your secret book about eternal youth

To understand what can go wrong and age you prematurely, it's necessary to know a bit about genes.

A genome, which consists of human genes, can be compared with a book. This book contains everything the body needs to know. It's written in a so-called "genetic" language. Each chapter contains unique stories (genes). Genes provide the codes for (for example) your intelligence, sense of logic and behaviour. The genes determine how our body and brain develop. We each have genes for memory and genes for our own unique ability to care, love and enjoy.

Genes you need to change

We also have some more unpleasant genes – those that contain codes for diseases: everything from chronic inflammation in the intestines to cancer, ageing and death. The genome, which I compared with a book, is very clever and can copy, read and repair itself. This is necessary, because it's not until the DNA string has been read, analysed and understood that it turns into a protein. Almost everything in your body is made from or because of proteins.

All cells contain DNA strings except red blood cells, egg cells and sperm cells. Your mitochondria (the part of your cells where energy is produced) also contain a DNA string. If there's damage to the DNA in your hereditary material, it will affect your entire body's energy production.

The enzymes that check for damage to the chromosome can be compared with an inspector in a workplace. If the inspector discovers a spelling mistake (damage to the gene), she'll try to correct it and prevent millions of defective copies from being made. Use the table below to identify the youth thieves that spoil the great work of your internal gene inspector.

Women, know your youth thieves. Make your food your burglar alarm and imprison all the thieves forever with your actions and your anti-ageing lifestyle.

Youth thieves that affect your biological age	Consequence	Symptom	Stop the youth thieves with
Exogenous/ endogenous stress	Destruction, oxidative stress	Inflammation, fatigue, poor detoxification, depression, hormonal problems, muscle fatigue and weak/low muscle mass	B9, B12, B6, magnesium, proteins, omega-3 fatty acids, vitamin C, coping strategies, music, wellness, therapy, coaching, self-love, and exercise
Free radicals	Oxidative stress, gene damage, DNA damage	Inflammation, wrinkles, sagging skin, and high blood pressure	Antioxidants, catechins such as green tea, pomegranates, blueberries, other berries, bioflavonoids, SOD (Glisodin), glutathione and Imedeen
Poor mitochondrial function	Oxidative stress, DNA damage and "fires" in your cells	Inflammation, disease, poor immune defence, hormonal problems, excess weight and obesity	Blood sugar stabilising food, proteins, omega-3 fatty acids, vitamins B1, B2, B3 and B5, magnesium, manganese, zinc, amino acids, Q10, exercise and muscle training
Lack of micronutrients	Gene damage, poor reading of the DNA, mutation, poor mitochondrial function	Disease, cancer, wrinkles, sagging skin and fatigue (including chronic fatigue)	Zinc, selenium, magnesium, manganese, iron, all types of vitamin B (six different types), biotin and vitamin C
Glycolysation ("caramelisation") of cells because of too much added sugar and starch	Oxidative stress, immune response	Inflammation, high blood pressure, high LDL, low HDL, excess weight and obesity, poor memory and concentration, Alzheimer's disease, dementia	Blood sugar stabilising food, proteins, omega-3 fatty acids, chromium, vitamins B1, B2, B3 and B5, magnesium, manganese, zinc, amino acids, Q10, green tea, exercise, muscle training, self-love, increased self-esteem, motivation techniques, coaching
Telomeres or the hour glass effect	Frequent cell division, oxidative stress	Premature ageing, cell death and inflammation	B6, B9, B12, antioxidants and green tea, omega-3, Astragalus, reservatrol

NOTE! Don't take any additional vitamins if you're already taking those described in chapters 5–7! You can see the list of supplements on www.pinetribe.com/thorbjorg/ supplements.

149

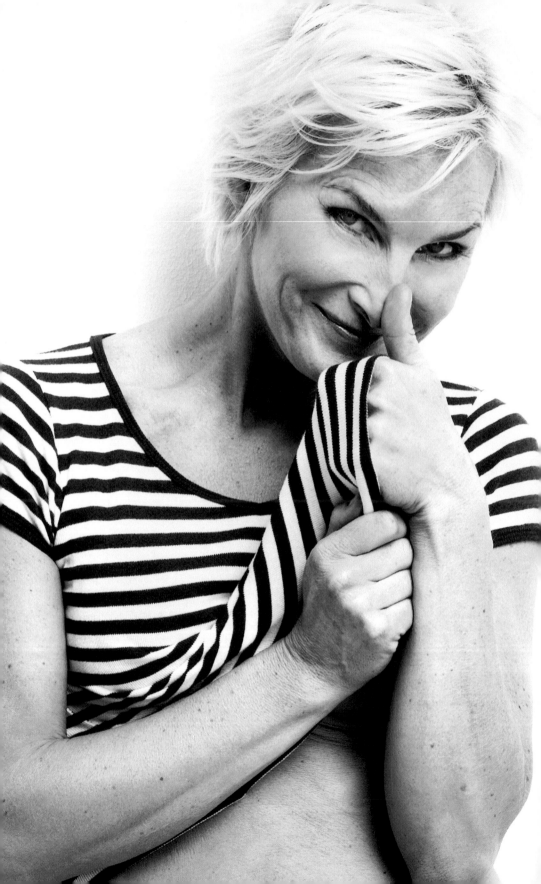

Lovely hormones instead of artificial ones

~~~~~~~~~~

No hot flushes or mood swings here

This week you're going to
- eat food and supplements that get rid of hot flushes, dryness (you know where), and mood swings.

You'll need
- good health food shops on the Internet or in your local area. See my recommendations throughout the book.

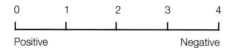

0   1   2   3   4

Positive   Negative

Each week you'll also need to write down what you have for breakfast, lunch and dinner every day. Don't forget to make a note of your snacks.

You can also see and fill out the table online at www.pinetribe.com/thorbjorg/my-charts

	Monday	Tuesday	Wednesday	Thursday	Friday	Saturday	Sunday
Energy 0–4 (describe)							
Digestion 0–4							
Bloating 0–4							
Weight							
Oedemas/swellings 0–4							
Headache 0–4							
Joint pain 0–4							
Muscle pains 0–4							
Bags/dark circles under your eyes/puffy eyelids 0–4							
Nose that runs/is congested 0–4							
Mucous in your airways 0–4							
Rash/eczema 0–4							
Dry skin 0–4							
Concentration 0–4							
Sugar cravings 0–4							
Mental state 0–4							
Feeling low 0–4							
Hormonal problems 0–4							
Irregular periods 0–4							
Hot flushes 0–4							
PMS 0–4							
PCOS 0–4							
Quality of sleep 0–4							
Exercise							

Supple hormones

I'm coming up to my 55th year and I've never felt better. Biologically, I'm 15 years younger. I'm going through a period of change that gives me the most amazing experiences and insights about myself and what I'm able to do. I've entered into a sacred pact with my hormones. They get what they need in terms of good food, healthy and friendly oils, the right nutrients and suitable loving care. In turn, I have no menopause symptoms – my gynaecologist says that the floor of my pelvis is firm and supple like that of a 20-year-old, my vagina is moist and I haven't lost my sex drive. I have no hot flushes or depression and I'm no more hysterical than I've always been! You can feel like that too. You can enter into that pact now!

Thorbjörg's six tips for a great hormonal system

1. Take 3 tbsp. cold-pressed flaxseed oil daily.
2. Eat 2–4 tbsp. ground flaxseeds and sesame seeds daily.
3. Use Estro Care body cream.
4. If you're over 40, take a quality menopause supplement from your local health food store or order online – see my recommendations on www.pinetribe.com/thorbjorg/womens-support
5. Exercise regularly.
6. Love yourself and give your needs priority.

Warning signs of hormonal problems
- Hot flushes
- Dryness
- Irritation
- PCOS
- Painful periods
- Reduced libido
- Irregular bleeding
- Depression
- Food cravings
- Mood swings
- Drama queen behaviour

Myth

Women stop producing hormones when they become menopausal.

Fact

Women never stop producing hormones. You can strengthen your natural balance by avoiding hormone-disturbing substances and filling your life with the right food, healthy fats, exercise, equilibrium and harmony.

Day 1

Test your hormones

Your own doctor or gynaecologist can measure what's called your hormone mirror. It's a good idea to ask your doctor to test your oestrogen, progesterone and testosterone levels. That'll tell you where you stand – whether you still produce enough hormones or are becoming perimenopausal. Note that the mirror only reflects a random day in your cycle. It doesn't give you a complete picture of how your cycle is "working".

I recommend you have a saliva test at a private laboratory instead. If you're still menstruating, you need to have your entire cycle tested, and it's necessary to collect test material throughout your menstrual cycle or for 28 days. That way, you can monitor a decline in oestrogen or progesterone levels. Afterwards, you can use targeted natural products to "tune" your hormonal symphony orchestra.

If you're menopausal and have stopped menstruating, you only need to test one single day.

It's also possible to test the relationship between the dangerous and the good oestrogen metabolites. Take the oestrogen test at www.pinetribe.com/thorbjorg/oestrogen-test. You can learn more about different hormone tests from your local functionally trained doctor (see www.functionalmedicine.org) who also can provide guidance according to your test results.

154

Day 2

Eat your way to harmonious hormones

Continue with your anti-ageing food from the previous weeks. It stimulates your hormone production and stabilises your blood sugar.

Let me repeat my food advice

Take organic, cold-pressed flaxseed oil every day, and eat fish three times a week and meat from animals that eat grass. Hormones need fats, so food low in fat is a catastrophe.

The cholesterol scare should be packed in a box and sent to the middle of nowhere. We need to produce cholesterol in order to make hormones. So get out your egg cups and your home-made mayonnaise. A bit of organic cream every now and then doesn't do us any harm either.

Remember

- Green tea
- Ground cinnamon
- Wholegrain products
- Fibre from beans and root vegetables
- Flaxseed oil
- Ground flaxseed
- The brassica cabbage family: broccoli, cauliflower, Brussels sprouts, white and red cabbage and radishes
- If you eat bread, make it rye and other food containing plant oestrogens (known as phytoestrogens)

Day 3

Balance hormones and blood sugar with food supplements

Melatonin is available on the Internet or from skilled treatment providers – take 3 mg per night for restless or poor sleep. Buy it from a good treatment provider or see www.pinetribe.com/thorbjorg/supplements.

- Lecithin granulate 1 tbsp. in your morning shake
- Vitamin B5 100 mg at night
- Vitamin C 1000 mg daily
- Chromium 200 µg 1–3 times daily with food
- Vitamin D3 (colicalciferol) 2000-4000 IU daily
- Magnesium citrate 400–600 mg daily
- Folic acid (B9) 1000 µg daily
- B12 (cobolamine) 1000 µg daily
- B6 100 mg daily

Always combine high dosages of individual vitamin Bs with vitamin B complex. See the Detox shopping list on page 103 for more information.

Day 4

Hormone-friendly natural products

A sugar-free lifestyle, low glycaemic food and good insulin sensitivity in your cells will protect you against cancer and help shift the oxidation of used oestrogens in the right direction.

Eat good fats, especially from flaxseed oil and ground flaxseed, as your hormones need the fat and lignans in the ground flaxseed. Take organic non-GMO soy milk and tofu in moderation, as the plant oestrogens balance your hormones.

Plants that support the oestrogen balance

- Red clover
- Liquorice root
- Angelica sinensis/Dong quai
- Indole-3-carbinols from the crucifer family: broccoli, cauliflower, Brussels sprouts and radishes
- Methyl donors/B12 and B9
- Green tea, which contains the very potent antioxidant EGCG (epigallocatechin-3-gallate)
- Black cohosh or black snakeweed is particularly good for hot flushes. See www.pinetribe.com/thorbjorg/cohosh
- Pomegranate juice and powder in capsules as supplements – a must. See www.pinetribe.com/thorbjorg/pomegranate
- Sage

Most of these are available at your local health food store or online. Check out www.pinetribe.com/thorbjorg/supplements for more information.

Why I choose the natural solution

When I was younger, I didn't want to challenge my body with the pill. And now, I don't want to give my body artificial hormones either. I don't dare disturb my natural hormone balance, challenge my detox abilities and risk breast cancer or blood clots in my legs (deep vein thrombosis).

Although my doctor says that oestrogen tablets can compensate when my natural hormone levels drop, I still don't dare. The fact is that the oestrogen I can get from my doctor is different from my own. And I don't want to give my body substances it doesn't recognise. Often, the doctor's oestrogens are made from premarin, which is urine from pregnant mares. The mare has already used them, detoxified them in its liver and excreted them in its urine, and then I am expected to use these sad remainders to help with my menopause. With my knowledge about the body and biochemistry, I say thanks, but no thanks to the mare.

Many women on my anti-ageing team confirm my concern. Premarin is broken down in a way that causes oxidative stress and binds with DNA and damages it. The result can be breast cancer (and prostate cancer in men).

Day 5

Drop hormone-disturbing factors from your life

- Avoid synthetic hormones and premarin.
- Avoid excess weight.
- Avoid excess alcohol, stop smoking and avoid passive smoking.
- Avoid soft plastic, especially plastic wrap in any form. It's a good idea to use glass containers for your food and leftovers.
- If you can, avoid food, oils, creams and lotions in plastic containers.
- Avoid pesticides (eat organic food).
- Avoid cosmetics and skin care products containing parabens.

Days 6–7

Hormone-friendly actions

- Exercise
- Relaxation – see week 8
- Healthy sleep, at least seven hours every night

Hurray for harmonious hormones

Oestrogen, progesterone and testosterone in the right balance keep you harmonious, happy, slim and young for longer, as harmonious hormones increase your insulin sensitivity, improve sugar metabolism, energy production and weight control and prevent premature ageing.

You can take active steps to avoid the female ailments and illnesses that relate to hormonal imbalance, nutrition and your body's communication.

- Osteoporosis
- Cervical cancer and cancer of the uterus
- Thyroid problems: hypothyroidism or hyperthyroidism (commonly called metabolic problems)
- Type 2 diabetes, syndrome X and obesity
- Breast cancer
- PCOS
- Stress and depression

You've now killed two birds with one stone. You live and eat in a way that keeps you young and helps your body tell your genes not to express cancer.

You now know that genes aren't static. You've been given the power to do something about them. Let's bust some more myths, while we're at it.

Useful geek knowledge about hormones

Our hormones are just like a symphony orchestra. If all the instruments are tuned and the conductor and the musicians are in good form, well rested, have had a good meal and agree about the score, nothing can really go wrong. Sweet music and harmony will fill the room and create an experience of calm, joy and energy. Your hormones are your instruments. You can tune them so they function optimally. What's their job and what tools do they need to work?

Hormones and their job

Hormones are chemical messengers that are released by an endocrine gland and transported in the blood.

Examples of endocrine glands

- The pancreas, which produces insulin, a blood sugar-regulating hormone.
- The thyroid gland, which produces metabolic hormones.
- Adrenal glands, which produce the stress hormones adrenalin and cortisol as well as the sex hormones oestrogen and progesterone.

Anti-ageing and anti-cancer lifestyle

Gorge on

- Cold-pressed, organic flaxseed oil.
- Ground flaxseed, organic quality.
- Cabbage from the brassica family: broccoli, cauliflower, Brussels sprouts, white and red cabbage.
- Chinese and red radishes.
- Red clover as a tea or supplement.
- Kuzu as a thickener (for sauces).
- Wholemeal rye in rye bread.
- Tofu and tempeh from soy beans.
- Isoflavones, genistein and daidzein from soy and tofu.
- Vitamins A, E (mixed tocopherols) and C in food and supplements.
- Alpha lipoic acid as a supplement.
  See www.pinetribe.com/thorbjorg/betaine
- Turmeric as a spice.
- Green tea. See www.pinetribe.com/thorbjorg/green-tea
- Lycopene from tomatoes (boiled or preserved).
- N-acetylcysteine (NAC) in food (onions, garlic, cabbage) and perhaps as a supplement. See www.pinetribe.com/thorbjorg/nac
- Low-glycaemic load food without added sugar.

Myths and facts about menopause

Myth

Hot flushes, excess weight, oedemas, grey hair, depression, raids on chocolate shops, murders of husbands and mental instability are the birthday present of women turning 45.

Fact

You can eat your way to healthy cycles, joy, fertility and regular periods until an advanced age. In the same way, you can avoid going grey too early.

Myth

Women under 30 don't need to worry about hormones, menopause, cancer or their age.

Fact

All women over 25 need to preserve their future beauty, firmness, vitality, health and youthful looks until an advanced age using my anti-ageing lifestyle. The earlier you begin, the more beautiful you will remain.

Scary examples

Early menopause caused by diet

Nina (aged 32) was one of my clients. She ate lots of white bread, sugar, white pasta and other high-glycaemic foods. Her blood sugar was in disarray and her body perceived Nina's poor food as information that triggered a major alarm. This alarm was registered in her brain, which sent out messages about the mess Nina was in via the pituitary gland to the adrenal glands. The adrenal glands react by producing the stress hormones adrenalin and cortisol. They raced out into the body with all lights flashing to reduce the consequences of this sugar alarm condition. But Nina was sugar-dependent so the situation was not just temporary and harmless. On the contrary, Nina was causing permanent damage to her body with the food she ate. Low insulin sensitivity, excess weight, inflammation, oxidative stress and "caramelising" of her cells were just some of the effects.

She was tired and off-colour, her mood fluctuated, she was quick-tempered, aggressive, and sad or depressed. She didn't sleep well, her muscles were sore and her periods irregular and painful. In addition to the hormones insulin, glucagon, adrenalin and cortisol, other hormones were becoming involved. You see, if one or more musicians in your hormonal symphony orchestra start playing out of tune, it affects the entire concert. Nina was not only in a chronic stress situation. Her sex and reproductive hormones were also seriously affected. Her oestrogens, progesterone and testosterone, menstrual cycle, regular periods and her ability to fall pregnant were in danger. She risked early menopause or a long and difficult menopause later on, with oedemas as an added bonus. The chronic stress Nina's body experienced could have had a negative effect on her metabolism and thyroid gland.

Food-induced hormonal disturbances

Another 43-year-old client called Jonna had long been overweight and afraid of eating fat. Name a diet and Jonna would have tried it. Years of weight fluctuations had left their mark on her body and biochemistry. Her brain was being bombarded with alarm signals.

- Too much sugar
- Not enough healthy fats
- Too much bad fat
- Too often hungry
- Too much bad food
- Blood sugar imbalance
- Insufficient and poor sleep
- Metabolic chemical substances and toxins from her liver and intestines
- Lack of self-confidence
- Lack of harmony

Jonna simply had too many defects in her genes. Her internal gene inspector wasn't getting the food and nutrition it needed to stop the defects and repair Jonna. She was insulin resistant and, in addition, the stress hormone cortisol was rushing through her body. Cortisol can be compared with a demolition firm that makes the muscles tired and weak. The skin becomes grey and sagging, and Jonna's thyroid gland and metabolism were under strain. She had too much testosterone in her body. Several years of imbalance between her oestrogens and progesterones had resulted in serious hormonal disturbances.

- Irregular periods
- Tender breasts
- Hot flushes
- Sweating
- Fatigue
- Feeling low
- Fibromyalgia-like symptoms
- Jonna is the "yoyo" exercise type

Young women in decline

It's not only women over 45 who become old before their time because of hormonal changes. I see too many women around 30 in my clinic with the same problems

- Excess weight
- Sweating and hot flushes
- PMS (premenstrual syndrome), irregular periods
- PCOS (polycystic ovary syndrome) and infertility
- Osteoporosis
- Reduced or non-existent libido
- High blood pressure
- Forgetfulness, difficulty concentrating and confusion
- Fear, anxiety and mood swings
- Sore and stiff joints
- Inflammation

163

- Tendency to bruise easily
- Wrinkles, dry skin and dry mucous membranes (vagina and eyes)
- Cell changes
- Breast cancer
- Fatigue
- Stress and strain
- Lack of energy and a desire to give up
- Emotional imbalance
- Difficulty sleeping

Women exposed to the food and lifestyle of the Western world are particularly likely to suffer from these symptoms. Until recently, Japanese women did not suffer from our common lifestyle-related illnesses such as cancer, cardiovascular diseases, type-2 diabetes, obesity and dementia. For thousands of years, Japanese women have eaten genuine food that the body can use and understand – tofu, tempeh, fish, vegetables and green tea.

Japanese women who moved to the West and eat Western food share all the diseases we struggle with here, which is a worry.

The good news is that Nina and Jonna changed their bodies and mental states by following my programme. You can also prevent early ageing and turn back the clock.

Healthy hormone harmony

This is why you need to eat your way to a healthy life
and oestrogen level

Oestrogens protect your beautiful bones and make them healthy. They also stimulate your breast glands, your uterus and your mucous membranes. Oestrogens caress the collagen in the subcutaneous tissue so it becomes elastic and firm without any major wrinkles. Oestrogen is also vital for the production of mucous in your vagina and throat, and the mucous membranes in your stomach, intestinal tract and eyes.

The oestrogen sends messages to your central nervous system to put you in a good mood, and provide good mental energy, libido, appetite, concentration and memory. The hormone keeps your heart healthy, your blood vessels in good shape and your blood pressure in balance. However, as with anything else in life, there has to be an equilibrium. Oestrogen is a hormone that stimulates growth for better or for worse. How can you get too much of it? You can if you get artificial hormones (in the form of the Pill or a hormone supplement, for example) and oestrogen-like hormones from the environment. A sudden drop in the oestrogen level or too much oestrogen in your body can cause breast cancer.

Hot flushes, anxiety, inability to cope, dry mucous membranes, reduced libido and irregular periods are warning signs that you should take seriously. Even if you're only about 30 years old.

This is why you need to eat your way to progesterone harmony

Just like oestrogen, progesterone affects your mental state and mood. You achieve a juicy sex life and well-functioning mucous membranes in your eyes and throat, etc. by creating a balance between progesterone and oestrogen.

An imbalance can cause anxiety, nervousness and a lack of energy – as well as dry mucous membranes, including in your stomach and intestinal tract. This causes digestive problems and a risk of infection.

Progesterone causes the cells in your ovaries and breast glands to mature. Harmonious progesterone is therefore your friend because immature cells can behave in a crazy manner, divide infinitely and become cancer cells.

This is why you need to eat your way to testosterone harmony

Sex drive, anger and the ability to express your innermost will are controlled by the male hormone testosterone. Men have plenty of this hormone, while we have to make do with it making up only 2% of our total sex hormones. But what a 2%! Testosterone builds and affects muscles, bones and the brain. It's the hormone that gives us drive and the courage to tackle new challenges. A balanced testosterone level promotes joy and mental energy, and keeps our fat production under control. It also controls both wanted and unwanted hair growth.

A lack of testosterone makes us weak, scrawny and unable to fight for ourselves and express our opinions. Hair growth on the upper lip, legs and back, as well as pimples and abscesses on the back and in the groin are unattractive signs of excess testosterone. The same applies to a deep voice and manly fat deposits on the stomach and waist, combined with thin legs. Women with these features are often insulin resistant (see chapter 4 about sugar).

Hormone harmony and a happy menopause

With all the knowledge you have now, there is no reason to fear the menopause. Look forward to it. It doesn't have to mean a loss of sex drive, beauty or vitality. You're the conductor of your own hormonal symphony orchestra. Soon, you'll know each individual instrument and the notes required to make sure your menopause is pure joy. It's not only your sex hormones that change during menopause. The entire symphony orchestra is affected when the musicians start playing a different tune. The following are some of the tunes that you have to pay attention to in your new life.

Challenge: a reduction in the human growth hormone (HGH)

The thyroid hormones TSH, T4 and T3, which affect your metabolism, slow down.

So does melatonin, which makes you drowsy and sleepy and guarantees good sleep –and is a potent antioxidant as well. The levels of the stress hormones adrenalin and cortisol in the body increase. This leads to a stress response and damage to the body. It can cause reduced insulin sensitivity in your cells, hair loss and loss of muscle mass, and can affect your central nervous system and your psyche.

Production of the hormone prolactin increases. Women sometimes experience this as inflammation, especially in their breasts.

This is what you do about it

Take melatonin as a food supplement. See www.pinetribe.com/thorbjorg/supplements.

Where do you find your healthy anti-ageing fats?

You can get healthy fats partly from animals that get the feed they are designed to eat, i.e. grass and unsprayed plants, and partly from some cold-pressed organic plant oils, like flax, pumpkin and olive.

Hormones in Hollywood

Women in the USA are lucky as they have doctors and specialists in women's health who use bioidentical hormones for menopausal women. Instead of synthetic progesterone, they use products such as progesterone cream based on natural progesterone-like substances derived from yams, an African root vegetable. They use plant oestrogens to support the oestrogen balance. If you're interested in learning more, you should read Suzanne Somers' book *The Sexy Years*. See www.pinetribe.com/thorbjorg/book-list

Fats as an anti-ageing miracle

10 good reasons to use healthy fats as an anti-ageing miracle

What you thought was the source of excess fat is actually the source of eternal youth. Fill your fridge with the anti-ageing remedy of the future – healthy, cold-pressed organic oils. Flaxseed oil, good quality fish oil and Udo's Choice (an organic blend of seed oils) are excellent examples of oils that will give you a beautiful body, harmonious hormones and silky skin, and make you burst with vitality. The following are 10 good reasons to drop the fat-free lifestyle.

1. A healthy production of hormones and a harmonious hormonal system without premenstrual problems, headaches, cramps and bad moods.
2. Superb metabolism and a constant weight. However, you will have to avoid starch, sugar, white bread, white rice and refined pasta. If you do, the fats in your body will ensure insulin sensitivity in your cells.

167

3. A loving heart that beats for yourself and your loved ones. Healthy, elastic blood vessels. Prevention of unhealthy layers of fat, poorly oxidised cholesterol and inflammation.
4. Good fat metabolism, a slim waist and flat stomach. Your body will have the courage to let go of its fat deposits when you give it vital fats in your food every day.
5. Healthy muscles, joints, mucous membranes and skin without inflammation, because omega-3 fats destroy inflammation.
6. Moist and well-functioning mucous membranes and therefore a good sex life. Flaxseed oil and fish oil in your food do wonders for controlling your oestrogen levels.
7. A superb immune defence. Your immune defence depends on good fats for fighting colds, flu and more serious diseases.
8. Good, healthy genes. Genes consist, among other things, of good fats, and your internal gene inspector needs omega-3 fats to successfully read the information in your genes and detect any damage. Damage to your genes can be caused by a lack of good fats.
9. Staying vitamin rich and vital forever. Many important vitamins are fat-soluble and can't be absorbed in your body without fats. You need vitamins for your immune function, hormonal system, blood quality and insulin sensitivity as well as for the prevention of osteoporosis, cancer, depression and cardiovascular diseases.
10. Clean throughout your life. Your liver needs healthy fats to detoxify your used hormones, environmental toxins, stress hormones and so on.

Therefore, eat:

- Organic chicken and game.
- Cold-pressed and organic flaxseed oil, thistle oil, hemp oil, sesame oil, olive oil and cold-pressed extra virgin coconut oil.
- Eat only organic butter that is not mixed with other oils.
- EPA and DHA: omega-3 fatty acids.
- Fish of all kinds, but especially fatty fish like wild salmon, ocean trout, herring, mackerel, sardines and tuna.
- Fish oil as a supplement.
- Cod liver oil.
- Alpha-linolenic acid: omega-3 fatty acids from cold-pressed, organic flaxseed oil.
- Ground, organic flaxseed.
- Linolenic acid: omega-6 fatty acids from cold pressed evening primrose oil, pumpkin seed oil and oil from nuts.
- Olive oil
- Almonds, hazelnuts, cashew nuts, walnuts, etc.
- Sunflower seeds, pumpkin seeds, sesame seeds, chia seeds– also ground or stored in their own oil
  - Almond butter
  - Tahini (sesame seed butter)
  - Peanut butter
- Omega-3 and omega-6 oils must never be heated under any circumstances.

Hormone-friendly beauty food

Top 3 hormone-friendly beauty foods

1. Proteins

You need proteins and their amino acids for your amazing cells, muscles, joints and skin, as well as for

- Stable controlled blood sugar levels.
- Increased energy.

- Better and more reliable weight control.
- Increased muscle mass and healthy cells.
- Good production of the antioxidants that keep you young and beautiful.
- Good detoxification.
- Alleviation of high blood pressure.
- Control of depression and melancholy due to low levels of serotonin and dopamine.
- The ability to manage stress.

Where do we find good proteins?
- Fish, lamb, poultry, game and eggs.
- Soy/tofu (contains plant oestrogens and inhibits inflammation).
- Pure whey protein powder.
- Brown rice protein powder.
- Hemp protein powder.
- Goat cheeses.
- Nuts, almonds, seeds and kernels contain L-arginine, which lowers high blood pressure.
- Pulses such as chickpeas, kidney beans, mung beans and lentils (not complete proteins, but contain a large number of the necessary amino acids).
- Spirulina.
- Chia seeds.
- Quinoa.

Avoid the unhealthy proteins
- Animals given feed they're not designed to eat.
- All food mixed with bad and unhealthy fat – tuna salad, prawn salad and other lunch salads.
- Salami and sausages made from animals given artificial feed and laced with colourants.
- Sliced processed meat that contains more than three additives or preservatives and is not organic.
- Sausage meat or meatballs with added starch and sugar.

- Minced fish products.
- Milk products with added sugar.
- Large amounts of milk and cheese.

2. Fibre

Fibre cleanses your intestinal tract. There are two types of fibre: those that are water-soluble and those that aren't.

Water-soluble fibre works like a vacuum cleaner in your intestines. It binds all the junk on the way to the toilet, for example hormones that have been detoxified in the liver and have worked their way through the gall bladder into the bowel. It also binds cholesterol and heavy metals. If hormones don't find fibre to hold on to, they can become "vagrants" in your system and find their way into your bloodstream. However, used hormones must be shown the door – they're no longer welcome in your body.

Where do we find good anti-ageing fibre?

- Root vegetables: sweet potatoes, carrots, beetroot, turnips, parsnips, celeriac, artichokes, Jerusalem artichokes and silver beet.
- Pulses: chickpeas, including hummus, kidney beans, mung beans, cannellini beans, adzuki beans and lentils, both green and red.
- Pectin from fruit, for example apples and pears.
- Ground flaxseed.
- Artichoke hearts.
- Don't forget psyllium husks, glucomannan / Konjac root or similar fibres.
- In addition to its ability to absorb liquid, fibre promotes good digestion and regular visits to the toilet.

3. Fruit and vegetables

The wow effect of fruit and vegetables cannot be overestimated. If we want to remain luscious for longer, our bodies must have delicious food. And it has to be green. Food that talks to the genes and keeps us as firm and juicy as the apples on the tree. That's what we have to eat. Anti-ageing food is fruit and greens. They give us fibre, antioxidants, phytochemical substances, vitamins, trace elements, vitality and great taste, all at the same time. Most vegetables are good anti-ageing food. However, phytochemical substances such as indole-3-carbinol help the liver get rid of used oestrogens and oestrogen-disturbing substances. That's why they're called cancer-preventing substances.

Where do we find good, hormone-friendly vegetables?

- Broccoli
- Cauliflower
- White and red cabbage
- Brussels sprouts
- Chinese and red radishes
- Lemon and lemon zest
- Orange and orange zest
- Grapefruit and grapefruit zest
- Watermelon
- Parsley and spinach
- Berries

Anti-ageing superfood

Eat some fruit, which is good for your hormones and helps you detox. Berries are the quintessential superfood, bursting with vitamin C and fibre. In addition, they're so gentle to your blood sugar that you can eat almost unlimited amounts without gaining weight. Go crazy with blueberries, strawberries, raspberries, blackberries, goji berries, and healthy cranberries.

The pomegranate is the oestrogens' best friend – it's full of ellagic acid, which appears to optimise oestrogens and stabilise typical menopausal problems. In addition, it tastes heavenly and looks beautiful in salads and desserts.

Fruit and berries are incredibly important and are wonderful for a sugar-free anti-ageing lifestyle. They beat the sweet taste from added sugar by miles.

Dried fruit is also fine, but has a higher glycaemic load than fresh fruit.

The hormonal effects of vegetables, fruit and berries
- Balanced hormones
- Effective detox
- Internal detox
- Better digestion
- More energy
- Stable insulin sensitivity
- Beautiful skin
- Better immune defence
- Improved concentration and wellbeing
- More effective protection against cancer

Avoid unhealthy fruit and vegetables
- Sprayed vegetables
- Tinned or frozen non-organic vegetables and fruit
- Vegetables baked in filo pastry
- Overcooked, "dead" vegetables
- Large amounts of potatoes
- French fries

WELL DONE! You've now completed my 10-week transformation
process. I congratulate you on your tremendous effort. It's time for
you to do the same. Pat yourself on the back, celebrate and acknowl-
edge your transformation.

Take the "Test your biological age" test again and complete the following form, just to remind yourself how amazing you are. If you forget later, you can always flick back and look at your pre-programme
photo and read how you felt at that time.

Biological age

How I feel physically

How I feel mentally

My daily diet

CHAPTER 11

Beauty: attractive skin throughout your life

~~~~~~~~~~

My skin hasn't changed much since I was in my 30s

You've now completed a transformation that will continue to have a huge impact on your wellbeing and health for the rest of your life. Do super anti-ageing skincare and skincare products help? Yes, they do, and even more so once you've completed the process that creates beauty and sex appeal from within. So let's celebrate your goodbye to the age of repair by taking a look at the amazing skin products and beauty routines that will keep your skin glowing for the rest of your life.

Fill your bathroom cupboard with pure, delicious, natural and fragrant treats for your skin. Hair colour, face creams and body lotion with ingredients mostly created by nature itself. Start by getting rid of all products with chemical formulas you don't understand in their list of ingredients. We don't want to spoil all your detox efforts by using hormone-disturbing substances.

Invitation to anti-ageing indulgence

Be happy! Four steps to celebrate your new looks.

1. Natural glowing skin

Start with your whole body. Scrub away the dead skin cells using a homemade body scrub. See www.pinetribe.com/thorbjorg/body-smoothie. Treat your skin with my fantastic homemade coconut oil with rose or lavender and smear it in – see the recipe later in this chapter.

Brilliant scrub using glycolic acid

Your skin will become incredibly smooth and beautiful with the following home beauty treatment. The honey contains glycolic acid, which is found in many anti-ageing exfoliants and wrinkle creams. It repairs skin cells and provides support to the collagen layer of the skin. It is when the collagen layer becomes loose that your skin starts wrinkling and sagging. Green tea is one of nature's most potent skin protectors.

- 25 g/ 1 oz fine oat flakes or almond flour.
- 1 tbsp. organic acacia honey.
- 1 tbsp. extra virgin coconut oil.
- ½ tea bag of green tea powder.
- Grind the oat flakes even finer using a blender or mortar.
- Mix the remaining ingredients with the fine oat flour.
- Clean your skin and pat it dry. Apply the mask and massage in small circular movements. Stand at your basin because flakes of the mask will fall off. Leave the mask on for 10–15 minutes. It stings, but that's OK, because it means that it's working.
- Wash off with lukewarm water and enjoy your "new" skin. Apply your favourite facial moisturiser afterwards.

2. Superb hair

Spoil yourself and make an appointment with your hairdresser. Preferably an organic hairdresser!

3. Soft feet

Make an appointment with a pedicurist and get soft, sexy feet. The mere thought of your well-cared-for feet will be a joy in itself.

4. Clean the slate

Make an appointment with a beautician and start your new life with deeply cleansed skin.

Thorbjörg's complete guide to skin indulgence

- Take skin-friendly food supplements such as SOD (Glisodin).
- Brush your skin with a bath brush every day.
- Exfoliate your skin twice a week.
- Use my homemade "AHA fruit mask" once a week.
- Always remove your make-up at night. Also use skin tonic, serum and perhaps night cream.
- Don't overdo sunbathing. Protect your head and face with an attractive hat or cap in summer.
- Prepare your skin before a holiday in the sun with natural tan optimiser and antioxidants. .
- Use a richer cream on your face in winter. Buy it online or at your local health food shop.
- See your beautician and have a facial once every six weeks.
- Pull faces and laugh a lot. It strengthens the connective tissue in your skin.
- Avoid puckered lines around your mouth by quitting cigarettes and drinking straws.
- Use a moisturiser when you travel by car, bus, train or plane. Use it generously and often.
- Drink lots of water.

- Make sure you get your vitamins and oils every day.
- Sleep well and for long enough.
- Eat nutritious and healthy anti-ageing food.
- Take supplements of vitamin D, colicalciferol 3, vitamins C and E and beta-carotene.
  See www.pinetribe.com/thorbjorg/supplements.
- Take silicium for beautiful skin, hair and nails.
- Drink plenty of green tea or take green tea in tablet form. See www.pinetribe.com/thorbjorg/green-tea.
- Drink unsweetened pomegranate juice.
- Avoid food that has been grilled for a long time.
- Avoid deep-fried food.
- Eat vegetables, fruit and berries in all the colours of the rainbow: watermelon, cantaloupe melons, spinach, rocket, parsley, blueberries, strawberries, raspberries, blackberries and the brassica cabbage family, which includes broccoli, cauliflower and white and red cabbage.
- Get rid of your wrinkles by eating cantaloupe melons!
- Eat sardines, salmon, shellfish, pulses and beans.
- Eat food that protects you against oxidative stress and damage in all the colours of the rainbow: fruit, berries, green tea and cabbage from the brassica family.
- Eat healthy fats in the form of flaxseed oil, evening primrose oil, fish oil and coconut oil (cold-pressed, virgin and organic).
- Eat food containing hyaluronic acid: root vegetables such as sweet potatoes, carrots and beetroot.

Dessert for your skin

Thorbjörg's exfoliating AHA mask for your skin. You can download it from www.pinetribe.com/thorbjorg/aha-mask

- 50 g / 1 ¾ oz defrosted berries
- ½ tea bag of green tea powder

Sieve the berries, mash them finely or blend them. Mix the green tea powder with the mashed berries. Apply the mixture to your face (take care to avoid your eyes) and leave the mask on for 10 minutes. Wash it off with lukewarm water and apply your favourite natural moisturiser.

Thorbjörg's ultimate skin products from top to toe

What works against wrinkles? What products are both effective and pure? What gives you beautiful hair and skin, a fragrant, pure and firm body without chemicals and nasty side effects? Below is a list of the products I always keep in my bathroom cupboard. They are listed from hair (top) to toe (bottom).

Be fussy about your products

There are millions of products on the market and I don't know all of them. Some anti-ageing products do what they promise and others do nothing at all. Check product ingredients and composition and the reliability of the manufacturer. The following is essential for me.

- The product must be organic or at least to a great extent.
- It should be free of parabens, damaged oils or other skin and hormone-disturbing substances.
- It should contain substances and compounds that are similar to those our skin is made of.
- It should contain antioxidants.

179

- It should contain moisturising substances.
- It should contain substances that support the skin's collagen and elastin.

Good brands
- Lavera
- Dr. Hauschka
- Jurlique
- Pure Deming
- Z. Bigatti
- Priori
- Ole Henriksen
- Dr. Alkaitis

Hair

Shampoo
The best
Logona shampoo and products are great as they contain nourishing proteins and oils.

Value for money
Velvet Rose from Sante is very good for my dry blonde hair.

Go to www.pinetribe.com/thorbjorg/shampoo for recommendations and information about a stockist in your area.

Conditioner

My favourite is Sante Brilliant Care Hair Conditioner. It contains nourishing oils and gives your hair volume instead of weighing it down and making it flat like many other organic conditioners do. See www.pinetribe.com/thorbjorg/conditioner

Hair treatment

The ultimate

Is your hair in need of therapy? Try out natural hair masks from different brands. Or try pure coconut oil or Moroccan argan oil. This is my favourite treatment because it keeps my hair looking nourished, moist and shiny. I use it once a week because my hair dries out quickly even though I use organic hair lightening products.

Good tip

The hair treatment can also be used for your skin – a couple of drops on your moist skin after a bath is enough.

Value for money

Use the same coconut oil you use for cooking. It must be cold-pressed, extra virgin and organic. I use mine after washing my hair and leave it for a couple of hours with my hair wrapped in a towel. It's good because the oleic acid nourishes and treats both hair and roots. Wash with a good shampoo applied to dry hair afterwards.

See www.pinetribe.com/thorbjorg/hair-treatment for recommendations and information about a stockist in your area.

Hair colour

I use a hair colour from Logona, which gives blonde and bleached hair a golden blonde look. Logona has many beautiful hair colours based on natural plant extracts, and the creamy products are excellent for covering grey hair. Go to www.pinetribe.com/thorbjorg/colour for information about a stockist in your area.

Styling

Wonderful

The John Masters Organics range of hair care products is my favourite. Bourbon Vanilla & Tangerine Hair Texturizer is a product made in heaven and I use it to style my hair. You only need to use a little in dry or wet hair and either leave your hair to dry naturally or use a hairdryer.

Indispensable

Sebastian crude clay. An earthy styling product based on clay. Available for approximately £26 / $45.

Hold

If I want my hair to look good all day long, or I'm going out in my little black sexy number at night, Natural Mist Herbal Hairspray is a safe bet. It's completely plastic-free unlike most other hairsprays.

Sante also produce an excellent hairspray.

Curls/body

Use Zenz Therapy conditioner when you've just washed and towel-dried your hair – don't rinse out.

See www.pinetribe.com/thorbjorg/styling for recommendations and to find a supplier.

Face

Creams

Luxurious

I have many favourites and I alternate between them.

Wonderful face mist NaþPCA from Twinlab. Great when travelling. Spray liberally and frequently.

There are various superb Antioxidant Face Creams available from different brands. Find one with the effective anti-ageing super antioxidant alpha lipoic acid, which is excellent for combating the impurities in the skin.

Clever

I also use pure Alpha Lipoic Acid Gel from The House of Deming, which I order online. I use it once or twice a week and it makes my skin soft, pure and glowing. It's superfood for your face, containing vitamin C, pomegranate, blueberries and other antioxidants.

Value for money
Lavera's Basis Sensitiv hand cream is only $16.95.

See www.pinetribe.com/thorbjorg/face-cream for this list of recommendations and suppliers.

Serum & Eyes

Luxurious
I use different kinds of serum. I make sure whichever kind I use contains hyaluronic acid and skinceuticals. You only need a couple of drops at a time.

Clever
Visage Ravissant Defy Damage from Beauté Pacifique is an effective anti-ageing serum that contains vitamin A and hyaluronic acid, which stimulates collagen growth. I also love using this product at night.

Anti-wrinkle
Dermalogica Intensive Eye Repair is superb against wrinkles. It's not cheap, but you get great value for money. It contains one nasty paraben substance, but I'm prepared to compromise because I love it so much. I trust that all the healthy food and antioxidants I consume ensure that my liver can neutralise a single "bad guy".

See a list of recommendations and suppliers on www.pinetribe.com/thorbjorg/serum

Facial cleansing

Cleanser/make-up remover and facial care
I use a very mild natural soap based on coconut oil for washing my face both morning and night. It's made by House of Deming and is suitable for all skin types. See www.pinetribe.con/thorbjorg/facial-cleanse for more information. You can also use pure cold-pressed coconut oil and a bit of cotton wool! Otherwise, you'll need a lot of water.

Exfoliate

Intense Mini-Peel from House of Deming with lactic acid or glycolic acid, which is also found in honey. See www.pinetribe.com/thorbjorg/exfoliate for more information.

After washing my face, I'm addicted to Lotion P50 1970. Actually it is my best secret. It's simply wonderful!

Value for money

For dead skin cells, I often use my own homemade oat and honey peel. It lives up to its reputation in Scandinavia, and is super-effective and cheap. See the recipe above. You can also try my AHA mask with berries – see the recipe earlier in this chapter. It's good for a slightly deeper peel.

Lips

Make sure to have it near you all the time, and that it's as simple and nourishing as possible. Otherwise it will just dry your lips out.

See my tips and recommendations on www.pinetribe.com/thorbjorg/lip-care

Tongue

A toothbrush and good oral hygiene are a must for me. However, my tongue scraper is just as important as my toothbrush. Every morning I scrape my tongue, and I can only encourage you to do the same with yours. Once you've tried it a couple of times, you'll understand

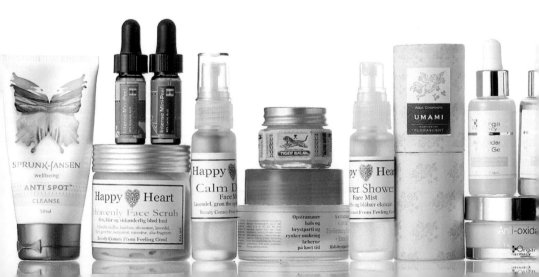

why. Get rid of the horrible whitish, greyish or greenish coating that attracts bacteria and bad breath. See www.pinetribe.com/thorbjorg/scraper for a list of suppliers.

Neck, chest and elbows

There is no reason not to use your face cream on your neck and chest as well. But your elbows need a richer cream. I treat them at night.

Hands

I tend to forget to use moisturiser on my hands, and I spend a lot of time cutting, peeling and rinsing vegetables as well as washing pots and pans. However, I try to remember to apply good, rich creams. Also I remember to use sunscreen on my hands every day.

See www.pinetribe.com/thorbjorg/hand-care for recommendations and information about a stockist in your area.

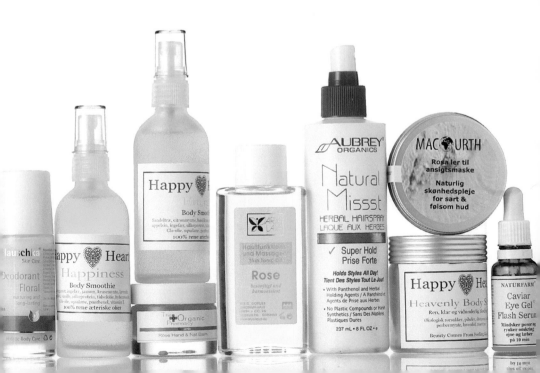

Your entire body

Soaps

Choose natural soaps based on natural oils and coconut. Liquid soap in bottles is also OK. See www.pinetribe.com/thorbjorg/soap for my recommendations.

Hair removal

Delicious

Moom with lavender for sensitive skin. It contains no irritating substances or synthetic perfume and lasts for a long time.

Value for money

The good old shaver. Use a rich soap that foams up well like shaving cream. I apply Traumeel from Heel cream afterwards.

See www.pinetribe.com/thorbjorg/hair-removal for my recommendations.

Cellulite

You've now mastered the diet and lifestyle that prevent and get rid of cellulite. The only other thing you'll need is a hemp glove and/or a soft skin brush.

See www.pinetribe.com/thorbjorg/anti-cellulite for more information.

The following is a very easy and effective weapon against cellulite and dead skin cells. Use it in your bath – then you can rinse off the salt, but don't use soap to wash off the oil because it should be allowed to work throughout the day.

- 200 ml cold-pressed extra virgin olive oil
- 80 g / 3 oz salt flakes, e.g. Maldon salt
- 1 tea bag of green tea powder
- ½ tsp. cayenne pepper
- 10 drops of aromatic pine wood oil

Mix everything together and store it in a jar with a lid. Massage in, using circular movements. Rinse the salt off in the shower and leave the rest to work throughout the day. You may need to use more salt. If so, just pour a bit of the oil over some salt in a small dish.

Body scrub

Delicious

When I'm in the mood for real luxury, I buy salt or sugar scrubs with natural organic oils and my favourite fragrance.

Value for money

Olive oil and salt flakes or brown sugar! I get a long way with that and my indispensable hemp glove.

See www.pinetribe.com/thorbjorg/bodyscrub for more information.

Body lotion

Extravagant

Firming Anti-ageing Body Cream. It detoxifies, cleanses and drains off unnecessary fluid. It's from The Organic Pharmacy and is very expensive. Or go for the natural solution from your local health food store, or make it easy and order your favourite online.

Fragrant

Basic moisturiser from Lavera is my favourite product because it smells good without being overpowering. It also really makes a difference to my skin.

Home-made

You can also use the homemade version with coconut oil and rose or lavender.

Go to www.pinetribe.com/thorbjorg/body-lotion for my recommendations and a list of suppliers.

Perfume and scent

Vanilla Oil is my "get in touch with your sensitive side" scent. I also really like the pure "Florascent" perfumes, especially those from Umami.

See www.pinetribe.com/thorbjorg/scent for more information.

Self-tanning

Self-tanning lotion from Lavera.

See www.pinetribe.com/thorbjorg/tan for a list of suppliers.

Sunscreen lotions

Remember to use them every day – all year round. Lavera anti-ageing SPF20 sunscreen lotion, Lavera anti-ageing face lotion, SPF15.

Natural sunscreen with factor 30, which can be bought online or at your local health food store. Go to www.pinetribe.com/thorbjorg/sunscreen for more information.

Feet

Epsom salts for foot baths and plenty of foot balm, which I massage into my feet until they are soft, warm and beautiful, see www.pinetribe.com/thorbjorg/footcare.

You don't need to spend all your money on luxurious and beautiful products.

Mix my homemade peeling masks, AHA acid mask, hair treatment and fragrant body oil, which you can find in this chapter. You can colour your hair in toxin-free colours yourself. You can also choose not to. You can choose a cheap, good face cream and spend money on the active substances Matrixyl 3000 and idebenone, which you can order online and add to your cream. They promote collagen growth and prevent wrinkles. See www.pinetribe.com/thorbjorg/anti-age for more information.

Woman, love your skin

Your skin breathes, senses, feels pain and protects you against the surrounding world. A bit of love and care is therefore appropriate for your largest organ. The skin consists of more or less the same material as your brain and peripheral nervous system. That's thought-provoking, isn't it? The skin serves as a kind of additional brain that perceives signals from within the body as well as from the surrounding world: pain, wellbeing, pressure, temperature, cold and heat. It's extremely good at asking your body to adjust to prevailing circumstances.

Your skin is also an important part of your immune system. Fascinating studies show how touch and massage benefit our health via our immune system, nervous system and digestive system. Your skin is your security guard. It protects you against foreign substances, wind and weather, pollution, excessive ultraviolet radiation, bacteria and viruses. Your skin has its own amazing flora of beneficial bacteria that contribute to this defence.

The skin produces vitamin D with the help of the sun's rays. Vitamin D is important for your immune system, your nervous system, the health of your bones and the insulin sensitivity of your cells. Your skin therefore contributes to keeping your bones healthy throughout your life, to a strong psyche free of depression, a stable weight and a wrinkle-free future.

Thorbjörg's own body oil with green tea

When I lived in Morocco many years ago, I learnt a trick from the young guys with bare torsos: to apply a mixture of olive oil and lemon juice to my body.

My version contains green tea, which protects the skin against the sun. Don't lie in the sun between 10 and 3, and use a high factor suntan lotion when you're in direct sun.

- 100 ml / ½ a cup cold-pressed extra virgin olive oil
- Juice of half a lemon
- 1 tea bag of green tea powder (www.pinetribe.com/thorbjorg/green-tea)
- A couple of drops of essential oil, either lemon or lavender

Place all ingredients in a clean empty bottle. Shake well and apply it to your body.

Thorbjörg's homemade coconut oil with rose or lavender

Melt 200 ml / 1 cup cold-pressed extra virgin coconut oil and mix with either rose or lavender essential oil. Put it in the fridge and let it solidify.

Now you're ready to fill your life with delicious products that are effective and add pleasure every day. Are you still finding it difficult to drop the expensive brands full of chemicals and hormone-disturbing substances, and instead invest in pure products? If so, it's time for some facts that'll make you fall in love with your skin and the good products that keep you beautiful at cellular level.

Your skin absorbs everything

Myth

Chemicals in creams are not as dangerous as chemicals in food. You don't eat them.

Fact

If the additives in your cream are small and fat-soluble, they penetrate the layers of your skin and enter your body.

Eat and be beautiful

Myth

Only suntan lotions keep your skin free of wrinkles.

Fact

Wrinkles on a woman have a lot to do with the amount of antioxidants, fats and low-glycaemic food she consumes. And whether she smokes of course!

Anti-wrinkle creams work

Myth

Anti-wrinkle creams are advertising rubbish.

Fact

It all depends on the ingredients and the reliability of the manufacturer. Some natural, pure active substances affect oxidative stress and wrinkles, and support the skin with the same the ingredients the skin is made of.

Did you ever get a big pimple on your face or a cold sore immediately before an important celebration or a performance that you were very nervous about? Or did you ever develop eczema or hives (urticaria) during a period when you were exposed to more stress than you were able to handle? It's no coincidence.

The skin is a barometer that shows how you feel. It gossips about what you eat, your feelings, your immune defence and your digestion. It exhibits your internal state. Hives and eczema are some of the symptoms exhibited by your skin when something is wrong, either emotionally or physically. Pimples and boils reveal nutritional and digestive connections. If your skin is very wrinkled, sallow, or loose, or lacks firmness and glow, this is a reflection of your lifestyle. It hasn't received the nutrition it needs, either because your food doesn't contain enough antioxidants, phytochemical substances and good fats or because you've had too much added sugar, too much stress, too much sun or not enough sleep and skin care. Or perhaps you've eaten well and healthily, but suffer from poor digestion and food absorption, or perhaps you smoke? A woman who has obtained a beautiful face and body through surgery, but still lives as she always did – unhealthily and without taking responsibility for her body – will never be as radiant as a woman with healthy skin and no other wrinkles than those that come naturally from smiling or laughing. A glowing and beautiful skin that is the picture of health shows that she is nutritionally and mentally balanced and that her digestion works as it should.

My youngest daughter, Telma Pil, who is 14, discovered the relationship between lifestyle and skin one Monday morning when she woke up with three ugly, infected pimples on her face. She'd been to the Tivoli Gardens with a girlfriend and they had been tempted by a "large revolting hot dog with all the ugly trimmings", as she expressed it. *Voilà!* Her skin revealed it right away. Good for Telma. At an age where pimples are everything – or rather avoiding them is everything – she learnt by experience and chose to act on it by deciding "I'll never eat that kind of junk again". Well done Telma, who decided early in her life to choose an anti-ageing lifestyle without being aware of it. She'll become aware of it later.

When I was Telma's age, I suffered from prurigo Besnier (atopic dermatitis), also known as infantile eczema. I had it on my face and neck and was really fed up with the large, red, very dry and itchy patches. I wasn't particularly well at that time of my life. I suffered from sugar dependency and had as yet undiscovered food sensitivities. In addition, or perhaps because of it, I had low self-esteem that clearly showed up on my skin. It took a few years, but they eventually disappeared entirely when I changed my eating habits, the way I perceived the world and my lifestyle in general. Later on it came back for a couple of years. The eczema and rash reappeared on my face, and I looked like a nightmare. I was wiser and knew from experience that my skin sensed what was happening in my life at the time. I was getting divorced from my husband of 25 years, and in addition, had a heavy workload at a new clinic and was working in a room with no windows and no fresh air. All these stress factors became too much and my immune system decided to remind me. In cases like this you have to act. Find a suitable psychologist or coach, change the room where you work and reduce your workload. You also have to help your body to get your immune response under control by taking the right supplements.

Anatomy of the skin

Your skin consists of several layers of epithelial tissue that protect the underlying muscles and organs.

The outer layer is called the epidermis and consists of the protein creatine and of melanin, which is responsible for pigmentation. The underlying layer is called the dermis and provides important support for the epidermis. The dermis contains

- Nerves and glands: oil glands and sweat glands.
- Hair follicles.
- Collagen, which is a supportive protein.

193

- Elastin, which is the flexible and elastic part of your skin.
- Lipids, such as glucosamines, which are sugar-like molecules that retain moisture in your skin.

Your skin can become seriously damaged by free radicals and oxidative stress, and it can undergo dramatic changes in health and appearance.

Do you remember the Ukrainian Victor Yushchenko, who was poisoned by his enemies a few years ago with dioxin? He survived, but his skin reflected the damage and oxidative stress the poison caused in his body.

The circumstances don't have to be that dramatic before oxidative stress damages your skin's ability to regenerate and repair.

- Collagen collapses and becomes loose.
- Elastin fibres become less elastic and slack.
- Lipids lose their ability to bind fluid, and your skin becomes dry and wrinkled.

Oxidative stress can be caused by

- Excessive sun tanning and sunburn.
- Photoageing (ageing due to exposure to UVA and UVB light).
- Smoking.
- Pollution and environmental toxins.
- Added sugar.
- Lack of good and healthy fats.
- Lack of micronutrients: vitamins and minerals.
- Lack of antioxidants.
- Lack of sleep and exercise.
- Lack of self-love.
- Stress.

To restore your healthy and young-looking skin, you need to treat and repair existing damage. If you follow my anti-ageing cleansing programme and my anti-ageing diet, your skin will improve dramatically. It is one thing is to eat the right food for healthy and wrinkle-free skin, but you also have to care for it from the outside. In principle, the products you apply to your skin should be so pure that you could eat them. However, there's one thing we have to look at first, and that's the sun.

The sun is your friend – but take care!

If you like sunbathing, it's imperative that you protect yourself against the sun's rays. They give you wrinkles and you could end up with skin cancer.

Get sun protection from your food

Make sure your skin is well nourished from within. It should have enough antioxidants, phytochemical substances, the right fats and liquid. Be sure to take

- Vitamin C.
- Vitamin E: as mixed tocopherols.
- Beta-carotene.
- EGCG and catechins from green tea.
- Superoxide dismutase – a "super killer" of nasties – and Glisodin (SOD).
- Alpha lipoic acid – a strong antioxidant that fights wrinkles from within.
- Anti-ageing food.
- Imedeen Tan Optimizer tablets.

Become beautiful with sun lotions

Use sun lotions that

- Are organic and plant-based.
- Have a high protection factor, at least 30 but preferably 50.
- Contain both UVB and UVA filters.
- Contain zinc oxide and/or titanium dioxide – the two substances that protect against the sun's rays - and nothing else. The lotions

MUST NOT contain parabens or other hormone-disturbing substances such as
- Methylparaben
- Ethylparaben
- Propylparaben
- Isopropylparaben
- Sodium methylparaben
- Butylparaben
- Isobutylparaben

Find the right sunscreen for you at www.pinetribe.com/thorbjorg/sunscreen.

Remember to use factor 15 for your face every day under your make-up. Sun damage (photoageing) occurs all year round. Sun protection is necessary, even if the sun isn't shining. Therefore, if you want to avoid wrinkles from sun damage, use sun protection every day.

On the beach, you should use at least factor 30 and apply it often and generously. It should be visible that you've used suntan lotion. That way you'll tan without causing sun damage to your skin.

DON'T lie in the sun between 10 and 3. It's a killer, whether you use suntan lotion or not.

Once your skin has become used to the sun, you can use my recipe for body oil with green tea described earlier in this chapter. It makes your skin beautiful and golden.

Super substances that are a must in your skin cream

When I shop for skin care products, I look for organic products that can strengthen collagen and elasticity, add moisture and prevent wrinkles. I insist that the products should be formulated based on scientific research and that the ingredients should be natural.

The following are the most important ingredients to look for when you read the labels

- **Matryxil 3000** is a peptide that activates, repairs and restructures your skin. It stimulates collagen and elastin-producing cells and makes your skin full and smooth. Clinical trials show an obvious improvement in coarse and rough skin, deep wrinkles and skin tone.
- **Ceramides** are lipids, similar to those we have in our cell membranes and brain tissue. They form protective tissue in the outer layers of the skin. Lipids provide moisture and reduce external exposure. It's the ability to retain moisture that makes your skin look youthful, glowing and full of vitality. We can thank the ceramides for that. The amount we have in our skin decreases with age and oxidative stress, and the skin can become dry, rough and wrinkled.
- **Coenzyme Q10** protects against damage to the outer layers of the skin. The amount of this enzyme in our skin decreases with age. Studies indicate an increased risk of skin cancer if the concentration of Co Q10 in the skin is low. Co Q10 is an important protective nutritional factor for the skin. It's a fat-soluble enzyme that you should take as a supplement and also apply via your skin care products.
- **Idebenone** is Q10's little sister. It's a much smaller molecule that's better at penetrating the skin. It's a very powerful antioxidant that repairs and strengthens the surrounding tissue, reduces fine wrinkles and makes you look younger. It protects against and reverses glycolysation in the cells – a form of "caramelisation" that occurs after prolonged excessive sugar intake.
- **Antioxidants** are extremely important for your skin. Pomegranates strengthen the anti-oxidative defence in your entire body and also support your hormone balance. They are an excellent ingredient in face creams. The cream's phenol content prolongs the life of your fibroblasts, which are the collagen- and elastin-producing cells in your skin. They also improve your skin's ability to heal after sun tanning and oxidative stress, protect you against skin cancer and inhibit inflammation.

- **Green tea** is undoubtedly the anti-ageing queen. Its polyphenol content is unsurpassed and fights oxidative stress and free radicals in your skin. It also repairs sun damage. It protects the DNA in your skin cells against ultraviolet rays (UVB rays). EGCG in green tea stimulates the growth of keratinocytes, which form proteins when applied to the skin – it becomes thicker, more resistant and robust. It also protects against skin cancer caused by oxidative damage from the sun.
- **Glycolic acid** has been on the market for a long time. It's a natural product extracted from sugar cane, fruit and honey. These sugar compounds are called AHA acids, of which alpha hydroxy acid is the most potent. They have a well-documented effect on the glow of your skin, the production of collagen and the breakdown of dead skin cells so that the skin appears healthy and smooth, full of vitality, alive and with a beautiful colour. It smoothes out fine wrinkles and protects against the sun's rays.
- **Hyaluronic acid** is also a large sugar-like molecule found in all the tissues in our bodies. It is particularly important for the tissue surrounding the cells in our skin. It binds with water and forms a gel-like substance that acts like a filler in our skin. smoothing out wrinkles. Hyaluronic acid is therefore important for the skin's moisture and structure. In addition, it stimulates wound healing and effectively protects against oxidative stress and damage.
- **Vitamins** are also good to have in creams, to protect against free radicals, smoke, sun, pollution and toxins. I especially look for the antioxidants vitamins C and E. The latter occurs naturally in the skin and is part of its immune defence. UV rays from the sun break down the vitamin E in our skin so it's necessary to apply it directly. The effect of vitamin C and the protection it provides against damage and the sun's rays are well documented. When it is applied to the skin, the sallow, yellow colour that can appear with age is toned down.

- **Alpha lipoic acid** is also a must for energy production and natural ageing. It counteracts and reverses glycolysation ("caramelisation") of skin cells. It must be in a form called R-ALA, a powerful antioxidant that repairs damage to skin cells and even damage to the DNA.

Fighting wrinkles

Fighting wrinkles with needles

The most commonly used substances for injections in the epidermis are Botox and Restylane. A qualified beautician, nurse or doctor injects the substance into the subcutaneous tissue using very fine needles to reduce both superficial and deep wrinkles.

The natural solution with needles

Restylane is made from hyaluronic acid, which is a sugar compound. It's the natural substance I mentioned earlier in this chapter, which is produced in all bodily tissue and acts by binding water. It does the same thing when injected into the skin – it binds water in the injected areas, and the gel-like substance formed acts as a filler in the injected areas of the skin, thereby smoothing out any wrinkles.

It has now been discovered that hyaluronic acid also stimulates collagen and elastin-producing cells.

The side effects of this treatment appear to be limited to irritation and reddening of the skin for a couple of days after treatment.

You can buy the hot, natural, skin-transforming substances Matrixyl 3000 and idebenone and add them to your own cream.

One of my absolute favourites is RejuveneX factor face cream. It contains almost all the things I want for my skin: Matrixyl, idebenone, pomegranate and green tea, R-ALA and vitamins.

Another favourite is Pure Vitamin Therapy, which is a wonderful, friendly and ethical product. It contains R-ALA (alpha lipoic acid) and pure vitamin C oil. The cream contains idebenone, green tea, vitamins and much more.

See www.pinetribe.com/thorbjorg/anti-age for more information.

The unnatural solution with needles

Botox is made from botulinum toxin A, which is a neurotoxin produced by the bacterium *Clostridium botulinum*. Botulinum toxin A binds two nerve endings and prevents the release of the neurotransmitter acetylcholine, which is necessary for muscle contractions. Many will be familiar with botulism – a serious infectious disease that causes death when the muscles in the airways or heart became paralysed. Why do people voluntarily choose to have botulinum injected into their bodies? Because it prevents muscle contractions and tension in the injected areas –and without them, no wrinkles.

Botox and possible side effects

- Dysphasia (lack of muscle contractions in the face, which can appear completely lifeless and without expression).
- Infection in the upper airways.
- Headache.
- Neck pain.
- Inflammation and sores at the injection site.
- Nausea.

- Personality changes.
- Asymmetrical facial expressions.

Botox has been used for medical purposes since the 1970s for the treatment of muscle tension and involuntary muscle spasms and so on. It wasn't until 2001 that it was approved by the American FDA to treat wrinkles.

Many face creams contain natural muscle-relaxing alternatives to Botox. Look for acetyl hexapeptide-3 and gamma amino butyl acid. The results are, of course, not as instant as with Botox – it takes several weeks to achieve the desired effect – but it lasts for as long as you use the product.

Natural facelift with massage

Without surgery and the risk that's always associated with skin intervention. It's also a lot less expensive. This massage can produce miracles. See www.pinetribe.com/thorbjorg/face-massage for recommendations and more information.

You'll receive compliments on your looks, which will be sweet music to your ears and your self-esteem. Accept it and enjoy it.

CHAPTER 12

Tips, tricks and survival guides

~~~~~~~~

You feel great in your new body. In fact, you feel better at every level – lighter, brighter and, in particular, younger in the right way. You have much more energy, you sleep better and perhaps you have started losing weight in a healthy and sustainable way.

This produces responses and reactions in your body, in your nervous system, and from your surroundings. You'll receive compliments on your looks, which will be sweet music to your ears and your self-esteem. Accept it and enjoy it.

Some people may see your new lifestyle and eating habits as a provocation and try to tempt you with cream cakes, marshmallows and words like "fanatic" or "health freak". An indulgent smile will sweep all these projections and envy out of your way. It's provocative to watch someone else stick to a healthy lifestyle, if you're unable to do it yourself. React with love and acceptance. It has nothing to do with you. Your inner voice, which was once very loud in its clamour for sugar, white bread or chocolate, could also raise its voice again. Before you tackle life as a changed woman, you need my tips for how to deal with relapses, kitchen frustrations and teething problems.

10 steps to prevent relapses

1. Never skip your breakfast and it MUST be rich in protein. The morning shake from the recipe section of this book is an excellent choice because it contains all the nutrients that will stabilise your blood sugar and remove your sugar cravings.

2. Don't underestimate your snacks. Your blood sugar needs some support throughout the day, and small snacks help. See the section on snacks in the recipe section of this book.

3. Eat protein for lunch. You need plenty of good vegetables and greens, but they aren't sufficient for your blood sugar. If you have sensitive blood sugar levels and tend to get tired, lose your concentration and energy, and are used to picking yourself up with coffee and chocolate, this is particularly important for you.

4. Don't keep any sweets, coke, sugar or food with added sugar in the house.

5. Never shop while hungry. You can be sure that you'll fill your trolley with all sorts of blood sugar-disturbing foods, which make you feel unwell and tired and give you a very bad conscience. It's not worth it. Therefore, do yourself a favour and shop on a full stomach, which means excess energy.

6. Always keep a rescue kit for your blood sugar in your handbag.

   - A packet of almonds.
   - A packet of almonds, raisins, goji berries and coconut flakes.
   - A packet of rye or buckwheat crispbread or rice biscuits, but eat only two at a time and always have some almonds or walnuts at the same time.
   - Fruit.
   - Carrots.
   - Dried fruit or unsweetened fruit and nut balls from your

local health food shop, or similar.

- Liquorice pastels (pure English liquorice without added sugar). See www.pinetribe.com/thorbjorg/liquorice
- A bottle of water or homemade green tea soft drink (see recipe in Chapter 13).

7. Don't forget your supplements.

- Take chromium tablets, 1–2 with food three times daily.
- Take green tea tablets.
- Take magnesium, 200–250 mg three times daily.
- Take omega-3 fish oil, 1000 mg.
- Add lecithin granulates to your shakes. See www.pinetribe. com/thorbjorg/lecithin for my recommendations.
- Use Bach Flower Essences and homeopathic products that support your process.

8. Drink water, at least 1½ litres (2½ pints) daily. When you get sugar cravings, start by drinking a large glass of water. It helps.

9. Make sure you exercise, preferably every day, if you're highly sugar-dependent.

10. Cheat your brain and talk it out of its sugar cravings. Talk in a way your brain understands: "I'm strong and can do without stimulants." or "I only eat food and sweets that are good for me and nourish me." In that way, you can consciously use your body's communication network to eliminate sugar cravings.

8 tips for bread lovers

1. If you pass a bakery on your way to work or school, then choose another route.
2. Comply with all the sugar prohibitions – they help in this case, too.
3. Eat a wholemeal bread roll or a slice of wholemeal bread very slowly and taste how healthy it is.
4. Try baking your own wholemeal rolls – that way, you'll get to know and love wholemeal flour.
5. Allow yourself one slice of white bread every weekend, if you think it's worth it. You'll quickly notice if you become tired, if your blood sugar drops, or if you get stomach ache, headache or aches and pains elsewhere in your body. If everything's OK, then just enjoy it.
6. When eating out, ask your waiter not to bring bread or ask them to remove it if it's already on the table. Otherwise, it's impossible to resist.
7. Imagine how the refined white junk sticks to your stomach and intestines. (It does!).
8. Imagine what the starch does to your blood sugar! (You know that from the chapter on sugar).

Survival guide for eating out

1. Choose good raw materials from the menu. There's always some fish or meat you can eat. Avoid sauces and melted cheese.
2. Choose plenty of vegetables and salad.
3. Avoid white rice. If white rice is part of the dish, ask the waiter to replace it with more vegetables.
4. Avoid white pasta and noodles. Ask to have them replaced with more vegetables.
5. Avoid bread and ask the waiter to remove it, if it's already on the table.
6. In general, choose fruit for dessert or maybe goat's cheese. If your blood sugar is under control, you can allow yourself something else every now and then.

7. Drink plenty of water during the meal.

8. If you drink wine, order a good one, preferably organic, and drink only 1 or 2 glasses.

9. Order green tea after the meal – it helps your blood sugar and digestion.

10. Remember to enjoy your meal.

Survival guide for travelling

If you're going to fly, take your own food, something like leftovers from your evening meal, or a salad with tuna or egg. You can normally buy good salads with egg, tuna or prawns at major airports. You can also often buy sushi, and if you do, don't worry about eating white rice for once. It's much better than what you can get on board the aeroplane. Bring almonds, raisins and vegetable sticks in your handbag. Remember to drink plenty of water and bring a couple of tea bags of green tea that you can dissolve in boiling water. That will save your trip. I never travel without a Greens powder. Ask your local health food shop to order some for you. It consists of freeze-dried vegetables, wheatgrass, barley grass and spirulina. You can also buy spirulina powder from your local health food shop or see www.pinetribe.com/thorbjorg/spirulina.

On my travels, I've always been able to find and eat anti-ageing food. It's all about eating pure raw materials and plenty of fruit and vegetables, and you can get that in most places. Choose your restaurants carefully or come prepared and investigate local conditions before you leave home.

In some countries, it's gradually becoming possible to buy rye bread, soy milk, rye crispbread, rice biscuits, plain (Greek) yoghurt, almonds and nuts, dried fruit and many other things that you need. Just look out for them at the local supermarket or grocer and you might get lucky.

You don't have to do without your protein shake, even if you stay at a hotel. Take your whey powder and a large shaker. Fill it with the powder, juice and water, give it a good shake and eat your fruit with the drink. You could also carry a hand blender and blend the whey powder with fresh berries and banana. If you have breakfast at the hotel, choose fresh fruit, plain yoghurt (if you can tolerate dairy products) and a boiled egg.

Kitchen tips and tricks

Kitchen tools that help you play around in the kitchen

1. A good blender. For many years, I've used my "lawn mower" with great success. It's a Vita Mix blender with a 2 hp motor. It can blend anything in no time. It even grinds chickpeas to chickpea flour! Check www.pinetribe.com/thorbjorg/appliances for some good recommendations. You can also check out what's available locally. KitchenAid is superb and Kenwood also works well. You can get small blenders with accessories at very reasonable prices. You can use them at home to grind seeds and they're also ideal to take with you on holiday. If you have one, you won't need an electric coffee grinder, which is otherwise a must for grinding nuts and flaxseed or other seeds.
2. A good kitchen appliance that can grate, cut, blend and knead. The Magimix food processor is fantastic if you enjoy cooking. However, a hand grater can also do the job.
3. Good pots made of steel or iron, but NOT aluminium or Teflon, which give off toxic vapours when heated.
4. A wok is a must for quickly frying vegetables or chicken. It doesn't have to be expensive, as long as it's made of iron or steel.
5. A steamer insert for your pots.
6. A clay pot or earthenware casserole dish is indispensable. Once you've learned how to use it and have experienced how good the food tastes, you won't be able to do without it. It's almost like having a chef employed in your kitchen.
7. An electric kettle for all the tea you drink!
8. A good teapot is nice for herbal teas and green tea leaves.

9. A juicer isn't a must, but if you'd like to make juice from freshly squeezed vegetables and fruit, you'll find a number of good brands on the market. Personally, I don't go for the most expensive model, as I prefer one that doesn't have too many parts to wash afterwards. Of course, the juicer must be able to squeeze the raw materials properly. See www.pinetribe.com/thorbjorg/juicer for my recommendations.

10. An electric coffee grinder for flaxseed and other seeds, kernels and spices.

11. It's very important to have good knives. Unfortunately, they're rare in otherwise well-equipped kitchens. You need different knives for different purposes, so a good set of knives is a good idea. They must be made of steel, always sharp and be stored in a knife block. Never wash them in your dishwasher – always by hand. Wash and dry them immediately after use. Good knives are like women: sharp, strong and to be treated with respect.

12. A vegetable peeler is indispensable for peeling fruit and vegetables, and making beautiful strips for your salads.

13. Use transparent glass containers for storage to avoid toxins from plastic getting to your food. Buy them in many different shapes and sizes. IKEA sometimes has some excellent glass containers that are stackable.

Flower essences can help, support and promote the body's understanding of changes. Choose 1–3 products.

Name	Characteristics	Use	Effect
Mimulus	Fear of letting go (old dependencies, e.g. sugar, bread, etc.)	2–4 drops directly on your tongue when the need arises	Genetic memory and communication network
Hornbeam	Fatigue, weakness, mental and physical exhaustion	4 drops directly on your tongue four times daily	Blood sugar, energy production and mitochondria
Aspen	Anxiety	4 drops directly on your tongue four times daily	Nervous system and neurotransmitter substances
Elm	Feelings of insufficiency and resistance to major challenges and responsibilities	4–6 drops directly on your tongue four times daily or 10–12 drops in water sipped throughout the day	Frozen nervous system and cell memory, communication network
Vervain	Overwork, stress, inner tension or excess enthusiasm	The same as for elm and can also be mixed with 6–7 drops of each	Communication network and adrenal glands
Ho-neysuckle	Living in the past, nostalgia, homesickness (old, unhealthy habits)	4 drops directly on your tongue four times daily or 10 drops mixed with mimulus in water sipped throughout the day	
Centaury	Lack of willpower, being easily influenced (by old dependencies)	4 drops directly on your tongue four times daily	
Rescue Remedy	Panic, anxiety, fear, fear of not living up to expectations	4 drops directly on your tongue when the need arises, but keep it in your handbag at all times	

Flower drops such as Bach Flower Essences are available from health food shops or can be purchased online. See www.pinetribe.com/thorbjorg/herbal-meds for more information.

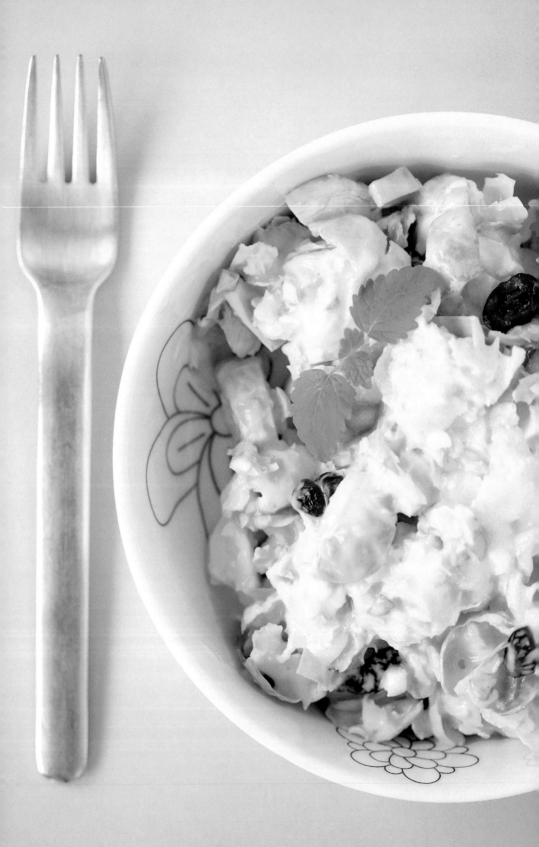

CHAPTER 13

Anti-ageing recipes

~~~~~~

My recipes make it easy for you to get started with your new anti-ageing lifestyle. I believe in a practical approach to cooking. Maximum benefit with minimum effort.

To enable you to use the recipes right away, I have prepared a weekly meal plan that will give you energy, power, flexibility, youthfulness and great flavours.

If your biological age is equal to or less than your age according to your birth certificate, you can eat more grain than indicated in this weekly meal plan. Your blood sugar will allow you to do so. You can eat more rye crispbread between meals, and it's also OK to use a little honey in your food or for your desserts every now and then.

If you're overweight and aiming to lose weight, I recommend that you go easy on the bread. Eat 1 slice per day and never two slices with the same meal.

Your body will now begin working seriously, using the food that promotes its healing capacity. It'll take time, and it's important that you give your body the necessary time. Don't just focus on your weight and get stressed about it. You'll lose weight eventually, anyway. First you'll notice signs that your body is responding to all the good things you're doing for it. You'll have increased energy, better sleep, fewer joint and muscle pains and better and more beautiful skin tone. Write it down. Keep track of everything that happens in your body for the next six months.

Weekly meal plan with super anti-ageing food

MEALS	Monday	Tuesday	Wednesday
Morning	Sexy morning smoothie (R)	Sexy morning smoothie (R)	Tofu shake (R)
Snack	Green tea, 10 almonds, 1 carrot	Fruit symphony (R), green tea	1 rice cake with almond butter, 1 orange, green tea
Lunch	Salad with the leftovers of Sunday's fried vegetables, sundried tomatoes, leafy green vegetables, ½ tin pulses, cold-pressed extra virgin olive oil and lemon juice	Salad (miscellaneous leafy greens), artichokes (jar), broccoli and chicken leftovers, almonds, canola oil, lemon and spices	Leftover radish salad with added tofu and Italian parsley, cold-pressed extra virgin olive oil and lemon
Snack	2 slices of rye or buckwheat crispbread with hummus (R), peanut butter, 1 carrot and green tea	1 slice pumpernickel bread or gluten-free bread with liver paté, a slice of baked beetroot, 1 cucumber and 1 carrot	Green smoothie with 2 tbsp. protein (R), 1 banana, 3 dates
Evening meal	Oven-roasted chicken (in earthenware casserole, if possible), root vegetable salsa (R), steamed sweet potatoes, broccoli and brown rice	Fish (salmon/cod), oven-baked for max. 12 minutes, a salad with fried radishes and barley (R), steamed cauliflower (2 minutes) with Ayurvedic ghee	Beetroot soup (R) with chicken pieces, 1 slice wholemeal bread or 1 home-made wholemeal spelt roll (R)
Evening snack	Watermelon, pineapple, mango or a bit of each, plus berries	Fruit with flaxseed mix (R)	Fruit and melon symphony (R)
Preparation	Soak whole barley in water with a few drops of apple cider vinegar or lemon juice. Prepare flaxseed mix for the whole week (R). Make a large portion of root vegetable salsa, so you have enough for a couple of meals. Bake beetroot, if you like it. Place whole beetroot in the oven in an ovenproof dish with water in the bottom for 90 minutes. You can use them the whole week as a side dish. Sweet, but without sugar! That's what we want!		If you wish, prepare the salmon burgers – it takes no time and they're better when stored overnight.

Thursday	Friday	Saturday	Sunday
Oat porridge with 1 tbsp. cold-pressed flaxseed oil, almonds, cinnamon, soy or rice milk, 1 egg	Sexy morning smoothie (R)	Tofu shake (R)	Brunch: Omelette with spinach (R), 1 wholemeal roll (R), soy latte
1 avocado with lemon juice, flaxseed mix, (see fruit symphony), green tea	2 celery or carrot sticks, 10 almonds, 1 pear, green tea	Lemon apples with flaxseed mix	Green tea and 10 almonds
Salad with tuna (tinned), egg and vegetables, sunflower seeds, ¼ tin kidney beans or mung beans, cold-pressed extra virgin olive oil	1 salmon burger (R), 1 tomato, shaved cucumber, 1 wholemeal roll with butter	Use sun salsa (R) as a basis for a prawn salad and spice it up with fresh coriander	Tomato soup (R)
2 slices of rye crispbread: 1 with herb paté and beetroot, and 1 with peanut butter and sliced boiled egg topped with cucumber and tomato, as well as berries	2 rice cakes or 2 slices of buckwheat crispbread with hummus (R) and chicken sausage, 1 carrot	1 slice pumpernickel bread with salmon (smoked or gravadlax) with pesto (R), 1 apple and a couple of figs	Gluten-free cinnamon cake bread (R), chai liquorice tea (R)
Salmon burger (R), sun salsa (R), warm tomato sauce (R) or 1 slice pumpernickel bread	Lasagne with goat's cheese and béchamel sauce made with rice milk (R), green salad with tomatoes, carrot sticks, beetroot sticks and red bell pepper, olive oil, balsamic vinegar, lemon juice and zest, basil	Rump roast (in earthenware casserole) with sweet potatoes, carrots and onions (R), boiled quinoa, rocket, cream and broccoli	Fried vegetables with leftover rump roast (R)
Apricots with goat's cheese and berries	Stewed fruit with oat milk and flaxseed mix (R)	Fruit symphony with cocoa powder and soy milk (R)	Cinnamon apple slices with walnuts, coated with coconut and wasabi
Prepare your own hummus (R), do so while preparing your evening meal. It's quick to prepare in a blender or food processor, but you can also buy it ready-made. Make a large portion of sun salsa (R), so you have enough for a couple of meals.	Write your shopping list for the weekend and the following week.	Prepare dough for rolls and leave to rise overnight (R). Make a lot and freeze some of them, so you have enough for the whole week.	Soak brown rice for 6–12 hours, add a couple of drops of apple cider vinegar or lemon juice. Soak almonds for 6–12 hours. Steam plenty of broccoli, so you have enough for the whole week.

215

Good advice for the detox programme in weeks 5–7

Everyday meals

1. Use the salad recipes below.
2. Boil fish for 3–5 minutes in lightly salted water OR
3. Bake fish in a pre-heated oven at 170ºC / 325ºF for max. 9 minutes (fillet or steak) OR
4. Fry in cold-pressed extra virgin coconut oil for 2–3 minutes on each side (see the salmon recipe).
5. Cut broccoli into florets and boil in plenty of water for max. 2 minutes. Prepare enough for several days and store in an airtight container in the fridge. Eat as required and add some to your salads.
6. You can do the same with cauliflower.

Prepare your own detox salad

1. Mix rocket, spinach, cos lettuce and parsley with broccoli or cauliflower. Add tomatoes, red bell peppers, prawns and pomegranate seeds, and use cold-pressed extra virgin olive oil, lemon juice, grated lemon zest, rosemary and garlic as dressing. Add a small amount of pepper and a touch of salt or tamari soy sauce to taste.
2. Use sun salsa or root vegetable salsa (recipes in this book) as the basis for your lunch or evening meal. You can add prawns, tofu, tuna or eggs, or eat it as an accompaniment to hot fish (fried, boiled or baked).

Recipes

Note: The recipes in this book show both British and American measurements, separated with a slash. For a list of equivalences see www.pinetribe.com/thorbjorg/measurements

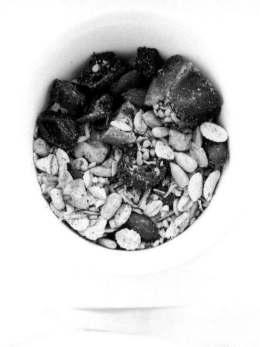

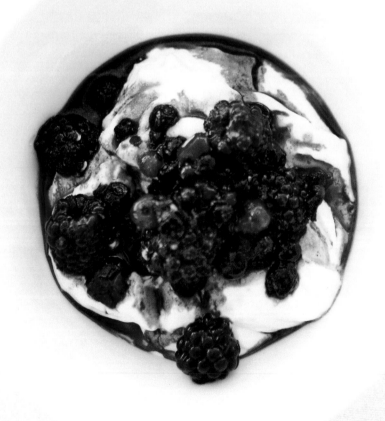

Breakfast & snacks

Detox shake
Serves 1

200 ml / 1 cup rice milk
2 measuring cups of
Fast And Be Clear powder
2 tbsp. cold-pressed virgin
flaxseed oil
200 g / 7 oz frozen berries
1 tsp. ground cinnamon
1 tbsp. lecithin granulate
Grated zest of 1 lemon
Blend all the ingredients together.

Green smoothie
Serves 2

Parsley is good because it contains glutathione, a so-called tripeptide. However, it also contains important vitamins and iron, which are incredibly important for preventing premature ageing. Parsley helps the kidneys restore the body's fluid balance. The parsley must be raw if all the healthy substances are to be preserved. The following is an extremely important green smoothie. If you drink it to quench your thirst, use half soy milk and half water. You can't eat too much parsley.

- 200 ml / 1 cup soy milk with calcium, rice milk or almond milk (available in most supermarkets) with 1 cm vanilla pod

- 1 large handful Italian parsley without stems
- 2 dried dates, pitted
- 4–6 ice cubes
- Place all ingredients in a good blender and mix at high speed. The parsley must blend with the liquid. You can add more ice and enjoy what it does for your fluid balance.

Dream on pink clouds
Serves 2

Watermelon. It contains something your fluid balance needs: a lot of water. The red colour is beta-carotene, which is the precursor of vitamin A. It also contains a powerful antioxidant called lycopene.

The clouds are there to keep your dreams in touch with reality! It's pure ying and yang. The egg whites deliver the protein we need.

- ½ (small) watermelon, peeled, white flesh removed
- 1 large handful fresh or frozen strawberries
- Juice and zest of 1 orange
- Juice and zest of ½ lemon
- 2 tsp. fresh rosemary, finely chopped

- 6–10 ice cubes, if you are using fresh strawberries
- 2 egg whites
- 2 tsp. xylitol (available from most health food shops)
- 1 tsp. liquorice root powder

Place all the ingredients except the egg whites and liquorice root powder in a blender and adjust the setting to high. If you want your drink a bit sweeter, you can add a couple of teaspoons of xylitol.

Whisk the egg whites with the liquorice root powder until stiff. They must be at room temperature, and the same applies to the bowl and the whisk.

Gently stir in the xylitol.

Serve in a large glass or a flat soup bowl with the clouds on top.

Sexy morning smoothie
Serves 1

Stabilises your blood sugar, talks to your genes and makes your cells happy. Enjoy it every morning. The amount of liquid and frozen berries determines the consistency. Sprinkle with femipower topping (see recipe for fruit symphony).

- 200 ml / 1 cup soy, rice or almond milk
- 2-3 tbsp. cold-pressed extra virgin flaxseed oil or Udo's Choice oil blend
- 1 tbsp. lecithin granulate, especially if you're stressed or have trouble sleeping
- ½–1 tsp. ground cinnamon
- tiny pinch of vanilla powder
- 1 tsp. grated lemon zest and a little juice
- 3 tbsp. pure whey protein powder
- 1 banana
- 150–200 g / 5-7 oz frozen berries

Blend all ingredients until the consistency is similar to a milkshake, yoghurt or soft ice cream.

You can play around with variations: orange zest and juice, fresh ginger, frozen banana, frozen mango or pawpaw, peanut butter, avocado, oat milk or pineapple. The most important thing is to have the basic ingredients: protein powder and oil. Whey protein can be replaced by rice protein powder, if available.

Tofu shake
Serves 2

- 1 ripe, but not overripe, avocado
- 100 g / 3 ½ oz silken tofu (available from most Asian shops or health food shops, and some supermarkets)
- 1 banana
- 1 tbsp. cold-pressed extra virgin flaxseed oil
- 200 ml / 1 cup rice milk
- 100 ml / ½ cup freshly squeezed orange juice or pure orange juice
- 1 cm vanilla pod

Place all ingredients in a blender and blend until the shake has a silky consistency. Then go ahead and enjoy!

Banana pancakes without gluten, milk or added sugar
Serves 3–4

- Leftover cooked brown rice or quinoa (350 – 450g / 1 ½ - 2 ½ cups)
- 3 eggs
- 100g / 1 scant cup buckwheat flour
- 100g / 1 scant cup quinoa flour
- 1 tsp. ground cinnamon (optional)
- ½ tsp. ground cardamom
- 2 mashed bananas
- 4 tsp. coconut oil

Mash the bananas and mix them with the eggs and melted oil. Mix all the other ingredients and gradually add to the wet mixture. The batter should be thick without being sticky. Cook in a hot frying pan with plenty of coconut oil or ghee – they should be the size of American pancakes. Eat them hot, plain or sprinkled with cinnamon, carob powder or blueberry jam without added sugar. Enjoy with a nice cup of green tea, cinnamon tea or chai with hot soy milk. Ideal with scrambled eggs to add protein to your breakfast. Otherwise, you'll feel like going straight back to bed afterwards.

Stomach-friendly muesli
Superb fibre for your stomach. It tastes so good that you might want to double the portion. Pure, healthy fats and blood sugar-stabilising cinnamon. Antioxidants from cocoa powder. A good dessert that will make your stomach happy.

- 325 g / 2 cups rolled gluten free oats or a mix of oats, rice and buckwheat flakes

- 60 g / ½ cup sunflower seeds
- 60 g / ½ cup sesame seeds
- 60 g / ½ cup pumpkin seeds
- 50 g / ½ cup almonds and walnuts, coarsely chopped
- 45 g / ½ cup coconut flakes, lightly roasted
- 10 g / ¼ cup dried cranberries or blueberries or goji berries
- 75 g / ½ cup raisins
- 30 g / ¼ cup dates, cut into 4
- 4 tbsp. cold-pressed extra virgin coconut oil
- 1 tbsp. pure cocoa powder
- 1 tbsp. ground cinnamon

Dry roast all the seeds in a frying pan, but be careful not to roast them for too long, or you'll damage the fats in the seeds.

Dry roast the rolled oats and/or other grains.

Dry roast the coconut flakes. Be very careful, as they quickly brown and burn.

Mix all the ingredients together. Mix in the coconut oil while the dry ingredients are hot. Store in an airtight container, preferably in a cool place.

Use muesli on plain organic yoghurt (if you can tolerate dairy products – otherwise you can use plain soy yoghurt) together with defrosted frozen blackberries/ mixed berries or fresh berries.

Morning porridge with quinoa or oats
Serves 3

Quinoa is the food of the gods – a protein-rich type of rice from Peru and Guatemala. The Incas considered it a gift from the gods because of its high nutritional value and pleasant sweet, nutty taste. This breakfast is low-glycaemic, rich in protein, tasty and quick to prepare.

- 70 g / ½ cup quinoa
- 200 ml / 1 cup water
- ½ tsp. salt
- 25 g / ¼ cup pear or apple, finely chopped
- 2 tbsp. raisins
- 30 g / ¼ cup soaked almonds
- 50 ml / ¼ cup rice milk or almond milk
- ½ tsp. ground cinnamon
- Toasted coconut flakes to sprinkle on top
- 2 tbsp. cold-pressed extra virgin flaxseed oil or good quality fish oil

- 2 tbsp. femipower topping to sprinkle on top (see recipe below)

Soak the quinoa overnight or for a few hours. Boil in the soaking water for 20 minutes before adding fruit, almonds and cinnamon powder and boiling for another 5 minutes.

Add the oil after arranging in a bowl.

Serve with rice milk or soy milk, flaked coconut, apple pieces and soaked sunflower seeds. Boil eggs and have with the porridge to make sure you get your morning share of protein.

You can use the same recipe with gluten free oats.
It's also an excellent bedtime por-ridge, especially good to prevent sleepless nights or restless sleep caused by unbalanced blood sugar and stress.

Fruit symphony

Cut apples or pears into large chunks or wedges and sprinkle with a little lemon juice. See below for a couple of variations to choose between. Eat with almonds or nuts, or coat the fruit with the following mixture:

Femipower topping

- 60 g / ½ cup flaxseed
- 60 g / ½ cup sesame seed
- 60 g / ½ cup hazelnuts
- 60 g / ½ cup almonds
- 1 tsp. ground cardamom
- 2 tsp. ground cinnamon
- 1 cm vanilla pod
- 1–2 tsp. liquorice root powder (if you like it)

Grind flaxseed and sesame seed in a blender with small blades that give a fine grind, or use an electric coffee grinder (inexpensive and important in this context).

Coarsely grind hazelnuts and almonds. Mix all ingredients together and store in the fridge, preferably in a dark glass container with a lid.

Use on your morning shake or sprinkle on your fruit snacks.

You can also sprinkle the following on your fruit

A bit of liquorice root powder or ground cinnamon, or carob powder with a little ground cardamom, or pure cocoa powder or wasabi powder.

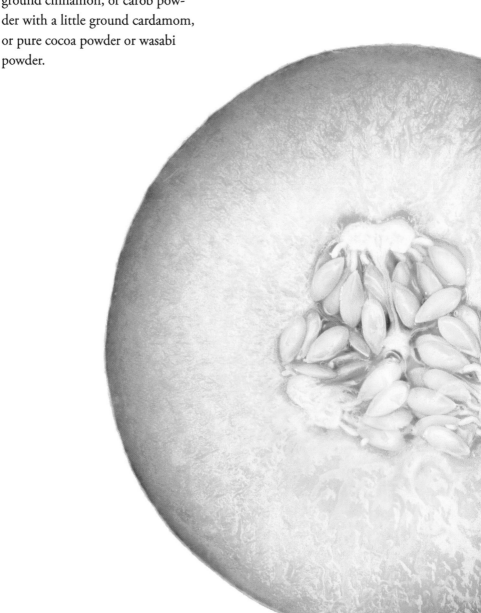

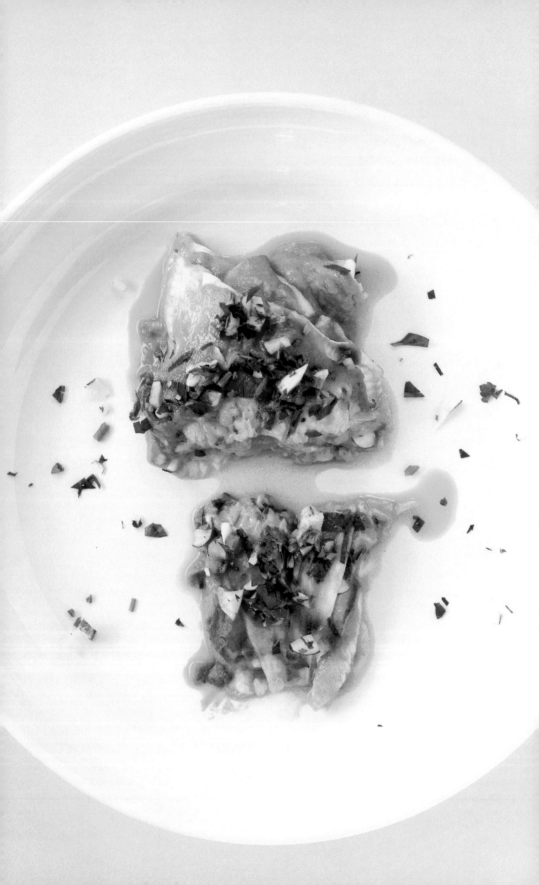

Lunch and evening meals

Bean salad with rosemary oil and garlic

Serves 2

- 1 tin borlotti or cannellini beans (the white ones) OR
- 160 g / 1 scant cup dried beans, soaked overnight in water and boiled for 1–1½ hours
- Approximately 20 fresh rosemary leaves OR
- ½ tbsp. dried rosemary
- 4 tbsp. cold-pressed extra virgin olive oil
- 2 garlic cloves, finely chopped
- Grated zest and juice of one lemon
- A little tamari sauce or other soy sauce
- 3 handfuls rocket or watercress

Drain the beans and place them in a bowl. Crush the rosemary in a mortar with a little olive oil and add to the beans along with the rest of the oil, garlic, lemon juice and zest. Immediately before serving, add the rocket or watercress.

Rump roast with soothing cloves

Serves 4–6

- 1 medium-sized veal rump
- 2 tbsp. whole cloves
- Sea salt and freshly ground black pepper
- 4–5 red onions, cut in quarters
- 500 ml / 1 pint water

You need an earthenware casserole or other ovenproof dish with a lid. Place the onions at the bottom. Rub the roast with salt and pepper and insert the cloves into the fat layer of the roast so it looks like a hedgehog. Place the roast on top of the onions. Add water. Cover and, if using an earthenware casserole, place in a cold oven and cook at 250°C / 480°F for 2–3 hours. The roast becomes incredibly tender, juicy and tasty. Use the stock to make gravy and thicken it with corn starch or rice flour. You can also use the stock to make soup. Serve with the onions.

Fish fillets
Serves 4

- 3–4 fillets of white fish from your fishmonger or frozen from the supermarket
- Juice of 1 lemon

Crumbing mix

- 75 g / ½ cup wholemeal spelt or buckwheat
- Sea salt and freshly ground black pepper
- 1 egg, beaten
- Butter and coconut oil, 1:1 for frying

Cut the fish fillets into suitable portions, sprinkle with lemon juice and store in the fridge overnight. Dip the fillets in the beaten egg and then in the wholemeal spelt mixed with salt and pepper. Fry for two minutes on each side in the butter and coconut oil.

Can be served with a dollop of mayonnaise. Mix the mayonnaise with Dijon mustard. It goes really well with the fish fillets.

Sun-baked chicken
Serves 3–4

- 1 chicken, organic or free range
- 1 orange
- 1 tsp. ground cinnamon
- 1 tsp. green tea powder (from your health food shop)
- Cold-pressed extra virgin coconut oil
- 1 green apple
- 75 g / 3 oz dried cranberries without added sugar
- Sea salt and freshly ground black pepper

Cut the orange into thin slices and insert them under the skin of the chicken. You can get access from both ends of the chicken: head and tail. Use a finger to loosen the skin on the chicken breast. Smooth out the orange slices and place them so they resemble a number of suns on either side of the backbone. Mix the cinnamon and green tea powder with 2 tbsp. coconut oil (leave the container on the kitchen bench or place it in a little hot water so it softens) and rub the chicken with the oil mixture.

Cut the apple into small pieces, and stuff the chicken with the apple pieces mixed with cranberries and a bit of cinnamon and green tea powder. Add a little salt and pepper. Place the chicken in an earthenware casserole. Add water so it half covers the chicken. Cover with a lid and place in a cold oven. Cook at 250ºC / 480ºFfor 1–1½ hours depending on size.

Choose a suitable salad to accompany the chicken and pour the stock from the casserole into small bowls and serve as soup.

Purple salmon
Serves 2

- 4 salmon steaks or fillets
- ½ tbsp. lavender (from your garden or a health food shop)
- 50 g / 2 oz blue poppy seeds

Green pesto

- 100 ml / ½ cup cold-pressed canola oil
- 1 bunch fresh coriander
- 1 slice dry wholemeal spelt bread
- Juice and zest of ½–1 lemon
- Juice and zest of ½ orange
- 1 cm vanilla pod
- Salt and freshly ground black pepper

Mix the salt and pepper with the blue poppy seeds and lavender.

Coat the salmon with the mixture and fry in cold-pressed extra virgin coconut oil.

Place the remaining ingredients in a blender and blend to a smooth, thick pesto. Serve the salmon pieces on a beautiful dish accompanied by the pesto.

Salmon burgers
Makes 4

- 2 salmon steaks (2 x 150 g / 5 oz) or 2 tins (2 x 210 g / 7 ½ oz) of salmon
- 1 egg
- 2 tbsp. lemon juice
- 1½ tbsp. Dijon mustard
- 2 spring onions or one small leek, finely chopped
- 100 g / ½ - ¾ cup oats
- A pinch of sea salt/salt flakes and freshly ground black or white pepper

Blend the oats finely in a blender. Set aside for later. Boil the salmon for max. 4 minutes in salted water and remove any skin and bones. Leave to cool OR drain the tinned salmon completely in a colander, then mix with mustard, lemon juice and onion in the blender.

Add the egg and mix thoroughly.
Add the oats last of all. Salt and
pepper to taste.

Leave the salmon mixture in the
fridge for one hour, or even better
overnight, before shaping it into
four burgers. Fry in cold-pressed
extra virgin coconut oil or half
butter and half olive oil.
You can also enjoy the salmon
burgers on a slice of wholemeal
bread with lettuce and slices of
tomato.

Prepare your own mayonnaise
2 egg yolks at room temperature
Approximately 100 ml / ½ cup
cold-pressed extra virgin olive oil
or canola oil (makes it sweeter)

Use a hand mixer or a whisk. The
trick is to mix a thin steady stream
of oil with the egg yolks while
whisking evenly until you achieve
the desired consistency. Add a
little lemon juice, Dijon mustard
or freshly ground pepper last of all
and serve with the salmon burgers.
Alternatively, buy organic mayonnaise from your health food shop
or supermarket.

Lasagna
Serves 4

- 500 g / 1 lb 2 oz minced veal
  or turkey – ask the butcher to
  mince it for you
- 1 large onion, finely sliced
- 1 large carrot, coarsely grated
- 1 red bell pepper, finely chopped
- 2 garlic cloves
- 2 tsp. dried thyme or marjoram
- 125 g / 4 ½ oz tomato concen-
  trate
- 1 tin peeled tomatoes
- 100 ml / ½ cup water

Wholemeal lasagne sheets OR alternatively two medium-sized zucchinis (courgettes) OR one large
zucchini cut lengthwise into thin
slices AND one mango, peeled and
cut into thin slices or strips.
A little salt and freshly ground
black or rose pepper or preferably a
pepper mixture, if you use minced
turkey.

Sauce

- 150–200 ml / ¾ cup water
- ½ tbsp. Plantaforce vegetable
  stock or similar quality stock
- Approximately 4 tbsp. brown
  rice flour
- 2 tbsp. coconut oil

- 85 g / 3 oz soft goat's cheese or soy cheese OR 100 ml / ½ cup oat milk
- 1 tsp. ground nutmeg
- 1 tsp. ground cinnamon
- Freshly ground pepper and a pinch of salt, but be careful if you use goat's cheese, as it's quite salty

Sauté the meat in the oil for a couple of minutes, then add onions, bell pepper and garlic, and sauté for a couple more minutes. Add the grated carrot and keep stirring. Add the spices, tinned tomatoes, water and tomato paste, mix thoroughly and leave to simmer on a low heat for as long as you can, but for at least 2–3 hours if you use beef or veal mince. If you use white meat, you will need less cooking time. However, the mixture must be well cooked and reduced – not a watery sauce, but full of flavour, so add a bit more of this and that if you think it needs it.

Prepare the sauce while the meat is simmering. Remember to pre-heat the oven to 180ºC / 350ºF. Bring the water and stock to the boil and set aside in a bowl.

Melt the oil in a saucepan and stir in the rice flour. Prepare a normal béchamel sauce by adding the stock bit by bit while stirring constantly. Take care NOT to burn the sauce. It must be smooth and not too thick – if necessary, dilute it with a little water. Add cinnamon, nutmeg and pepper to taste. Add the cheese last of all, remove the saucepan from the heat, cover and leave the cheese to melt into the sauce for a few minutes. Mix everything together. If you don't use cheese, add the oat milk or soy cheese when finished.

In an ovenproof dish, place layers of meat, sauce and either lasagne sheets or zucchinis and mango and then another layer of meat, sauce and zucchinis and mango, making sure you finish with a layer of meat and sauce on top. The layers can be mixed together a little bit.

Bake in a pre-heated oven for 30 minutes.

Warm tomato sauce
Serves 2–4

- 1 medium-sized red onion, finely chopped
- 1 red bell pepper, seeded and finely chopped
- 4 tomatoes, seeded and cut into wedges (alternatively one tin of diced, peeled tomatoes)
- 2 celery sticks, finely sliced
- 2 garlic cloves
- 200 ml / 1 cup orange juice without added sugar or freshly squeezed
- 1 tsp. oregano or thyme
- Sea salt and freshly ground pepper

Sauté onions in half cold-pressed extra virgin olive oil and half butter. Continue to sauté, adding the bell pepper and a bit later the tomatoes, orange juice and spices. Leave to simmer for half an hour. Blend the sauce in a blender and return to the saucepan. Add more water or orange juice if the sauce is too thick. Add celery and let the sauce boil for a couple of minutes before serving. Goes well with salmon burgers, as well as chicken and turkey, or as a pasta sauce served with wholemeal spelt pasta or soba (buckwheat noodles).

Omelette with spinach
Serves 4

- 4–6 large eggs
- 100 ml / ½ cup oat or soy milk (available at most supermarkets but alternatively, you can use rice milk)
- ¼ tsp. ground nutmeg or freshly grated nutmeg
- 2 tbsp. grated parmesan or soy parmesan
- 2 handfuls spinach leaves, alternatively defrosted frozen spinach
- A pinch of salt and freshly ground black pepper
- A little butter or good quality cold-pressed extra virgin coconut oil without coconut flavour for frying, or use a ratio of 1:1

Whisk eggs, oat milk and nutmeg in a bowl and fry in the oil in the frying pan over moderate heat. Add the spinach and use a spoon to gently push it into the egg mixture, when it is starting to firm up. Add salt and pepper to taste. Turn the omelette using a spatula and fry on the other side until light and golden. Can be served with melon for brunch.

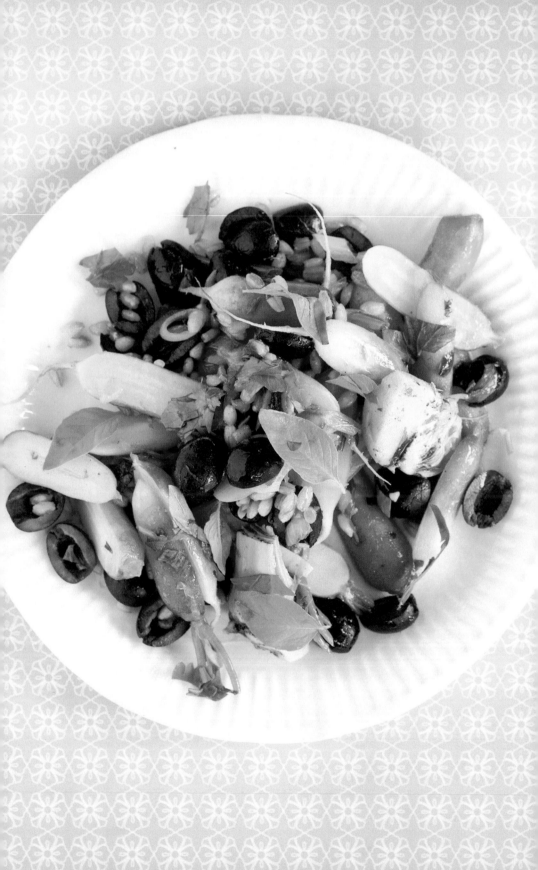

Vegetables, salads & dressings

Adzuki beans with grapes and olives
Serves 2

- 150 g / 1 cup dried or 1 tin adzuki beans or other beans, e.g. kidney beans
- 40 g / ½ cup green olives, pitted and cut in half lengthwise
- 80 g / 1 cup black grapes, seedless or halved and seeded
- 2 tbsp. cold-pressed extra virgin olive oil
- 1 tbsp. cold-pressed extra virgin flaxseed oil
- 1 tbsp. tamari soy sauce
- 1 tbsp. lemon juice and finely grated zest of ½ lemon
- 1 red chilli cut into fine strips
- Salt and freshly ground black pepper
- 1 bunch watercress
- Some borage flowers for decoration (optional)

If you use dried beans, soak them overnight. Boil them for at least one hour. Drain and cool. If you use tinned beans, drain off the liquid. Mix the following in a bowl: oils, soy sauce, lemon juice, salt and pepper. Add olives and grapes together with the beans, toss in the dressing and leave the salad to stand for a while. Add the watercress gently immediately before serving and decorate with borage flowers.

Broccoli and tofu salad
Serves 2–4

A really woman-friendly salad!
- 1 small head of broccoli
- 1 small red onion
- 1 apple
- Almonds that have been soaked in water overnight
- ½ handful raisins
- Tofu marinated in a little orange juice, fresh ginger and tamari soy sauce

Salad dressing
- 3 tbsp. cold-pressed extra virgin canola oil
- 1 tbsp. lemon juice
- A little balsamic vinegar
- A pinch of salt
- 1 cm vanilla pod
- ½ tsp. ground cinnamon
- Salt
- Freshly ground black pepper

Remove the stem of the broccoli immediately below the head. Cut into small florets. Cut the stem into thin slices, but remove the stringy outer layer. Steam the florets in a saucepan with steamer insert for max. 3 minutes, or boil in plenty of boiling water. Keep your eye on the clock. The broccoli should be *al dente* and crisp. When steamed sufficiently, cool in cold water and place the florets into a bowl.

Cut the tofu into cubes and place in a bowl. Sprinkle with soy sauce, orange juice and fresh ginger. Use approximately 1 tbsp. finely chopped ginger. Preferably prepare the marinade the night before so the tofu has time to absorb the flavours.

You can now do the following: either steam the tofu for 10 minutes in a saucepan with a steamer insert, BUT make sure it is placed in a bowl or on a plate, OR place the bowl with the tofu in a saucepan with water in the bottom and boil for 10 minutes, covered, OR toss the tofu in olive oil or coconut oil until the chunks are smooth and delicious.

Cut the onion into rings. Cut the apple into thin, half-moon-shaped wedges. Place in a bowl or a container if you plan to take it to work. Remember the almonds.

Pour the salad dressing over and toss immediately before serving. Add salt and pepper to taste.

Fiery fibre with beans
Serves 2

- 3 handfuls baby spinach
- ½ medium-sized bulb of fennel cut into paper-thin slices – use a vegetable slicer or mandolin
- ½–1 tin kidney beans, chickpeas or other pulses
- ½ jar sun-dried tomatoes in cold-pressed extra virgin olive oil
- 1 carrot, thinly sliced with a potato peeler
- 4 tbsp. cold-pressed extra virgin olive oil
- 1 garlic clove
- 2 tbsp. lemon juice and finely grated zest of ½ lemon
- 1 tbsp. balsamic vinegar
- ½ tsp. ground cinnamon
- 2–3 tbsp. roasted pumpkin seeds
- Salt and pepper

Mix all ingredients in a bowl and enjoy!

Pomegranate and celery salad
Serves 3

- 1 medium-sized ripe pomegranate
- 1 apple, thinly sliced
- 1 small handful of walnuts, coarsely chopped or halved
- 2 large handfuls of green leaves:

baby spinach, rocket, basil, parsley, mint and/or lemon balm
- 1 celery stick, finely sliced
- A handful of strawberries, halved lengthwise (leave out if not in season)
- Juice and grated zest of 1 orange
- 4 tbsp. cold-pressed extra virgin canola oil
- 1 cm vanilla pod
- A pinch of salt and freshly ground black pepper

Remove the pomegranate seeds from the fruit. Place the seeds and all the other ingredients in a large salad bowl.

Mix the oil and orange juice, whisk and pour over the salad immediately before serving.

Hummus
Serves 2–4

- 210 g / 1 ¼ cups boiled or tinned chickpeas
- 2 garlic cloves
- Juice and grated zest of ½ lemon
- 2 large tbsp. tahini (available from supermarkets and health food shops)
- Salt
- Freshly ground black pepper
- 1 tsp. ground cumin

Place all ingredients in a food processor or a good blender and mix until you achieve a silky consistency. The perfect snack. You can also use hummus as a spread on wholemeal crispbread, gluten-free crispbread or rice biscuits.

NOTE! Soak dried chickpeas in plenty of water for 12 hours. Boil for 1–1½ hours until tender.

Tinned chickpeas are available from many supermarkets and most health food shops. Watch out for added sugar, which should, of course, be avoided.

Warm radish salad
Serves 2

- 170 g / 1 cup buckwheat groats or whole barley
- 2–4 artichoke hearts in cold-pressed extra virgin olive oil
- 40 g / ½ cup black olives, halved
- 2 bunches of radishes
- 1 chilli, seeded if you prefer it less spicy, and very thinly sliced
- Grated zest of ½ lemon
- Sea salt and freshly ground black pepper
- A small handful of finely chopped Italian parsley

- Cold-pressed extra virgin coconut oil for frying

Soak the buckwheat/barley in water for a few hours with a little lemon juice or vinegar. Boil in the water used for soaking for 20–25 minutes. Add a little salt.

Place the cooked buckwheat/barley in a bowl.

Remove the green tops of the radishes and cut them in half lengthwise. Fry them in coconut oil for a couple of minutes together with the olives. Mix the radishes and all the other ingredients with the buckwheat and add salt and pepper to taste. Sprinkle the parsley over the warm salad immediately before serving.

Paella with quinoa
Serves 2–4

- 150 g / 1 cup quinoa
- 800 ml / 3 ½ cups water
- 1 tsp. turmeric
- A pinch or a couple of threads of saffron
- Cold-pressed extra virgin olive oil and coconut oil for frying
- 1 zucchini (courgette), cut into thin strips lengthwise with a vegetable peeler
- ½ bulb fennel, in fine strips (use the half left over from the beetroot soup)
- 1 red bell pepper, cut into long thin strips lengthwise
- Salt and freshly ground pepper
- ½ tsp. fennel seeds
- 300 g / 10 ½ oz frozen prawns
- 1 garlic clove, peeled and finely chopped
- Juice and zest of ½ an organic lemon

Defrost the prawns. Fry them for half a minute on each side in olive oil and garlic, place on a plate and sprinkle with a little lemon juice.

Dry roast quinoa grain in a saucepan while stirring until it begins to pop. Add the water and bring to the boil. Turn down the heat, cover and leave to simmer for 25 minutes until soft but not mushy.

Keep an eye on the quinoa. Take care that it doesn't burn or stick. Add a little olive oil when the water has almost completely evaporated. Add the olive oil and coconut oil to a frying pan. Add the vegetables and sauté with the spices until

239

tender (but not too soft). Set them aside for later.

Add a bit more oil to the frying pan, fry the turmeric in the oil and toss the quinoa in the oil until golden. Place in a dish, topped with vegetables and prawns, add the rest of the lemon juice and decorate with lemon zest.

Root vegetable dip
Serves 4

- 1 celeriac, peeled and cut into medium-sized chunks
- 1 medium-sized carrot
- 1 large red onion or 2–3 spring onions, finely chopped
- 2 medium-sized OR 1 large sweet potato, peeled and finely chopped
- 140 g / ½ cup tomato paste
- 1 tin peeled and chopped tomatoes
- 2 garlic cloves, peeled and finely chopped
- 200 ml / 1 cup freshly squeezed orange juice or orange juice without added sugar
- Grated zest of 1 orange
- ½–1 red chilli with or without seeds (very hot with seeds!), finely chopped (take care not to get chilli in your eyes!)
- ½ tbsp. dried or fresh oregano
- ½ tsp. grated nutmeg
- 1 cm vanilla pod
- A little cold-pressed extra virgin olive oil for frying

Sauté onions, garlic and root vegetables in a little cold-pressed extra virgin olive oil. Add the peeled tomatoes, orange juice, tomato paste and spices, and leave to simmer for at least half an hour.

Place everything in a blender and allow to cool before blending until you achieve a creamy consistency. Add salt to taste and perhaps a bit more vanilla. The cream should be spicy and sweet.

Serve warm or cold with cold meat or fish OR use as a vegetable dip.

Root vegetable salsa
Serves 2–4

- 2 small OR 1 large sweet potato, peeled and finely diced
- 1 carrot, scraped and finely diced
- 1 mango, peeled and finely diced
- 40 g / ½ cup black olives, halved lengthwise
- 60 g / ½ cup raisins that have been soaked in water

- 1 red bell pepper, cut into long strips
- 1 red chilli, with or without seeds, cut into fine strips (take care not to get chilli in your eyes!)
- 1 tbsp. lemon juice
- 1 tbsp. apple cider vinegar
- 50 ml orange juice, freshly squeezed or unsweetened
- 1 cm vanilla pod
- A handful of chopped Italian parsley

Boil sweet potato, carrot and red bell pepper in water for max. 2 minutes. Drain the water, place the vegetables in a colander, and cool under running water.

Carefully drain off all water before placing the vegetables in a bowl and adding the remaining ingredients. The salsa tastes even better if you leave it to stand for a couple of hours.

Serve with fish or white meat. Can also be made into a prawn salad by adding defrosted cooked prawns or prawns in brine as a lunch dish or starter. It also tastes heavenly with avocado.

Brussels sprouts in heavenly mango cream
Serves 3

- 400 g / 14 oz Brussels sprouts, finely chopped in a food processor or by hand
- 2 oranges, peeled, all the white pith removed and then sliced
- 75 g / 3 oz dried cranberries or raisins

Mango cream

- 1 ripe mango, peeled and finely diced
- 6–8 tbsp. cold-pressed extra virgin canola oil
- 3–4 tbsp. lemon juice
- Sea salt flakes
- 1 cm vanilla pod

Mix everything in a blender until the consistency is soft and creamy. Mix the cream with the Brussels sprouts. Can be prepared the day before, as the taste improves if left to stand.

You can also use the cream for fruit salads and to accompany cold meat. Keeps for a couple of days in the fridge in an airtight container.

Beetroot soup
Serves 4

- 1 medium-sized beetroot, peeled and cut into sticks
- 1 large carrot, scraped and sliced
- 1 medium-sized red onion, peeled, halved and sliced
- 1 small fennel bulb, finely sliced or cut with a mandolin
- 1 large garlic clove
- 4 fresh sprigs of thyme OR 2 heaped tsp. dried thyme
- ½ tsp. ground cinnamon
- 1 tsp. cumin
- 2 bay leaves
- 1 tsp. fennel seeds
- 1 tbsp. Herbamare vegetable stock or similar
- 1–2 tsp. sea salt, e.g. Maldon
- 750 ml / 3 cups water
- ½ jar (100 g / 3 ½ oz) concentrated organic tomato paste

Topping
- Soft goat's cheese

Sauté all vegetables except fennel in cold-pressed extra virgin olive oil and add all the dry spices. Add the water a bit at a time together with the vegetable stock and mix well.

Leave the soup to simmer for 15–20 minutes, then add the tomato paste and the finely sliced fennel. Add salt and freshly ground pepper to taste or a little chilli or cayenne pepper. Cook for another 2–3 minutes.

Top each portion with a couple of tsp. goat's cheese and serve hot. Goes well with a slice of wholemeal bread and butter.

Sun salsa
Serves 2–4

Remember to have the salsa with protein. Prawns go really well with this dish.

- 70 g / ½ cup whole quinoa
- 75 g / 3 oz dried cranberries without added sugar
- 2 garlic cloves, finely chopped
- 50 ml / ½ cup cold-pressed extra virgin olive oil
- 1 red onion, finely diced
- 1 zucchini (courgette), finely diced
- Juice and zest of ½ lemon
- Juice of ½ orange
- 1 cm vanilla pod
- 1 tbsp. finely grated ginger
- 5 tsp. tamari soy sauce
- 2 pinches cayenne pepper

Dry roast the quinoa in a saucepan for a couple of minutes.

Add 200–300 ml / approx. 1 cup cold water and boil for 20 minutes.

Keep an eye on the quinoa to prevent it from burning. The grains should not be too soft. Set aside and leave to cool. Mix the remaining ingredients and add the cold quinoa. Leave to stand for a couple of hours, preferably overnight, before serving.

Goes well with chicken, fish or salmon burgers (see recipe).

Spring cabbage with oat milk
Serves 4

- 1 whole head of spring cabbage
- 200 ml / 1 cup oat milk (available from some supermarkets, or alternatively use soy milk)
- 1 tsp. nutmeg
- Salt and pepper

Bring 1½ litres / 6 ½ cups of water to the boil. In the meantime, cut the whole head of spring cabbage into fine strips.

Toss it into the boiling water and cook for max. 2 minutes. Keep an eye on the clock. Drain the cabbage in a colander. Return the cabbage to the saucepan.

Add the oat milk, nutmeg and perhaps a dollop of butter. Add salt and freshly ground black pepper to taste. Add 1 tbsp. maize flour or rice flour to thicken. The cabbage is now ready to serve.

Spinach with wasabi
Serves 4

- 4 handfuls baby spinach
- 50 ml / ¼ cup cold-pressed extra virgin canola oil
- 100 g / 3 ½ oz walnuts
- 1 generous tbsp. cold-pressed extra virgin coconut oil
- ½ tbsp. acacia honey
- 1 tbsp. wasabi powder (available at most supermarkets or in Japanese shops)
- 75 g / 3 oz blue cheese (if you can tolerate cheese)

Start by briefly dry roasting the walnuts in a frying pan. Add coconut oil and roast for another 30 seconds. Add honey and stir. Add the wasabi powder and toss well. Remove from the frying pan and leave to cool. Enjoy as a snack or as an accompaniment to a meal.

Place the spinach in a salad bowl together with the blue cheese cut into small chunks. Pour the oil over the spinach and add as many walnuts as you like. Goes well with fish, chicken or game.

Tofu salad
Serves 2

- 2 tbsp. cold-pressed extra virgin coconut oil
- 2 cm fresh ginger cut into thin strips
- 1 garlic clove
- 100 g / 3 ½ oz broccoli in florets, boiled for one minute in plenty of lightly salted water
- 2–3 asparagus spears: cut off the tops, halve the stems once lengthwise and chop in half. Boil for one minute with the broccoli.
- ½ endive (chicory), stalk removed and coarsely chopped
- A couple of fresh spinach leaves, preferably the coarse ones, not baby spinach
- 100 g / 3 ½ oz tofu
- 1 tbsp. water
- 2 tbsp. wheat-free tamari
- 2 tsp. roasted peanuts, sunflower seeds or pine nuts

Heat the oil in a frying pan or a wok. Toss garlic and ginger in the oil. Add all vegetables as well as tofu, water and tamari. Stir over high heat until the vegetables are tender, but not soft.

Serve with toasted nuts or seeds and perhaps a bit of fresh coriander on top. It's OK to eat a slice of wholemeal rye or spelt bread with the salad.

Tomato soup à la the legendary Campbell's
Serves 4

- 750 ml / 3 cups passata
- 70 g / ¼ cup concentrated tomato paste
- 400 ml / 1 ¾ cups coconut milk
- ½ tsp. nutmeg
- Salt and freshly ground black pepper

Put the passata and tomato paste in a saucepan and bring to the boil.

Add the coconut milk and nutmeg, and salt and pepper to taste.

That's all there is to it, and it tastes sooooo good! It's a good idea to add protein in the form of a tin of kidney beans without added sugar (discard the liquid) or a handful of prawns together with a slice of wholemeal bread and butter.

Rolls & bread

~~~~~~~~

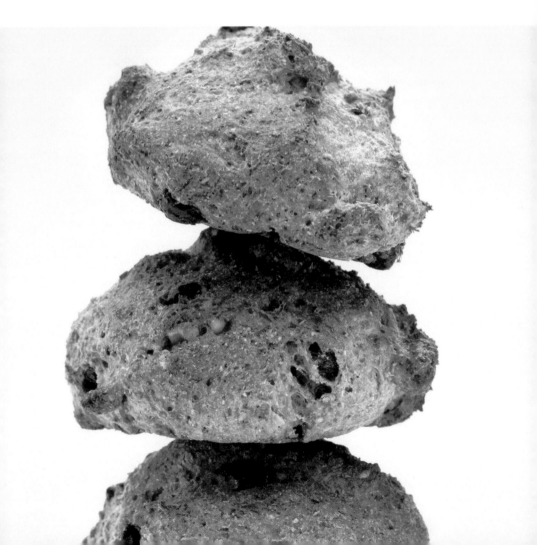

Wholemeal spelt bread

You can quickly convert this recipe to rolls. No rising time required, but the bread improves if left to rise overnight.

- 750 ml / 3 cups lukewarm water
- 1 sachet dried yeast
- 2 tbsp. honey
- ½ tbsp. salt flakes or coarse sea salt
- 150 g / 5 oz coarsely chopped hazelnuts
- 125 g / 1 cup raisins
- 60 g / ½ cup sunflower seeds
- Approx. 300 g / 10 ½ oz finely ground wholemeal spelt flour
- Approx. 500 g / 1 lb 2 oz coarsely ground wholemeal spelt flour

Mix the yeast, salt and honey with water. Add the nuts, raisins and seeds and leave to soak for 10 minutes.

Carefully add the finely ground flour first and then the coarsely ground flour bit by bit. Mix until well combined and you can't stir any more. This dough doesn't require kneading and shouldn't be too dry. Divide the dough and place into two baking tins. Bake in a 180ºC /350ºF pre-heated oven for 45 minutes.

You can bake the dough as rolls instead, and the baking time is then 25–30 minutes. Keep an eye on them.

Gluten-free wholemeal rolls
Makes 8

- 500 ml / 2 cups rice milk or soy milk
- 30 g / ¼ cup psyllium husks
- 250 g / 9 oz cornflour
- 100 g / 3 ½ oz buckwheat groats
- 75 g / 3 oz brown rice flour
- 50 g / 2 oz butter or cold-pressed extra virgin coconut oil
- 25 g / 1 oz fresh yeast
- 1 tsp. salt
- ½ tsp. ground coriander
- ½ tsp. ground fennel

Mix the dough with an electric mixer. Heat the milk until lukewarm and place in the mixing bowl together with the psyllium husks. Mix for five minutes until it forms a gel-like substance. Mix the flour, butter, crumbled yeast and spices in a separate bowl before adding to the milk and psyllium mixture and stirring for 15 minutes. Cover the mixing bowl with plastic wrap and leave to rise in a warm place for 30 minutes.

Smear a little oil on your hands before handling the dough. Knock the air out of the dough with a fist. Remove enough dough for one roll with a spoon and roll into a sausage shape with your hands. Place the rolls upright like small towers on a baking tray lined with baking paper and cover with a moist tea towel. Leave to rise in a warm place for ½–1 hour.

Brush with the soy/rice milk.

Bake at 250ºC / 480ºF for 10–20 minutes.

Gluten-free cinnamon cake bread

Tastes great, also good with butter.

- 50 g / 2 oz ground sesame seeds
- 150 g / 5 oz brown rice flour
- 150 g / 5 oz buckwheat flour
- 100 g ground hazelnuts
- 100 g / 3 ½ oz rice flakes
- 2 tsp. ground cinnamon
- 2 tsp. ground ginger
- 2 tsp. ground cloves
- 1 tsp. ground cardamom
- 1 tsp. nutmeg
- 1 cm vanilla pod
- 3 tbsp. carob powder or cocoa powder (optional)
- 1 tsp. salt
- ½ tsp. black pepper
- Juice and zest of 1 orange
- 125 g / 1 cup raisins or coarsely chopped dates
- 2 tsp. gluten-free baking powder
- 100 g / 3 ½ oz cold-pressed extra virgin coconut oil
- 4 bananas
- 2 eggs

Mix the bananas, coconut oil and eggs in a food processor or electric mixer. (Alternatively, you can mix everything by hand.) Add the orange juice.

Mix all the dry ingredients in a bowl and add bit by bit to the wet banana mixture while stirring.

Pour the dough into a greased baking tin (or tins) and bake at 180ºC / 350ºF in a pre-heated oven for 45 minutes. Leave to cool before slicing.

Gluten-free flaxseed bread

- 170 g / 6 oz flaxseeds
- 1 litre / 4 ¼ cups water
- 30 g / ¼ cup psyllium husks
- 200 g / 7 oz buckwheat groats
- 340 g / 12 oz millet flakes
- 230 g / 8 oz buckwheat flour
- 100 g / 3 ½ oz cornflour

- 120 g / 4 ½ oz brown rice flour
- 30 g / 1 oz honey
- 25 g / a scant 1 oz carob powder
- 2 tsp. salt
- 2 tsp. ground coriander
- 2 tsp. dried oregano

Mix the dough with an electric mixer. Grind the flaxseed finely (use an electric coffee grinder or a blender with small blades). Heat the water until lukewarm and place in the mixing bowl together with the psyllium husks. Mix for five minutes until it forms a gel-like substance. Mix the flours, honey, carob and spices in a separate bowl. Add to the bowl with the psyllium husks and stir for 15 minutes. Grease a baking tin (3.3 litres / 3 ½ quart) or line with baking paper greased with butter or coconut oil and pour the dough into the tin. Brush the surface with oil and cover the tin with aluminium foil. Shape the foil like a lid so it covers the sides of the tin. Leave the bread in a warm place (approximately 28ºC / 82ºF) for 24 hours until it has risen above the edge of the tin. Place the bread with the foil in a cold oven on the bottom shelf.

Bake at 175ºC / 350ºF for 2 hours 10 minutes with the foil – and another 10 minutes without the foil. Leave the bread in the tin for 10 minutes before turning it out and wrapping it in a moist tea towel to stand until the following day. Can be sliced and frozen.

For your sweet tooth

~~~~~~~~

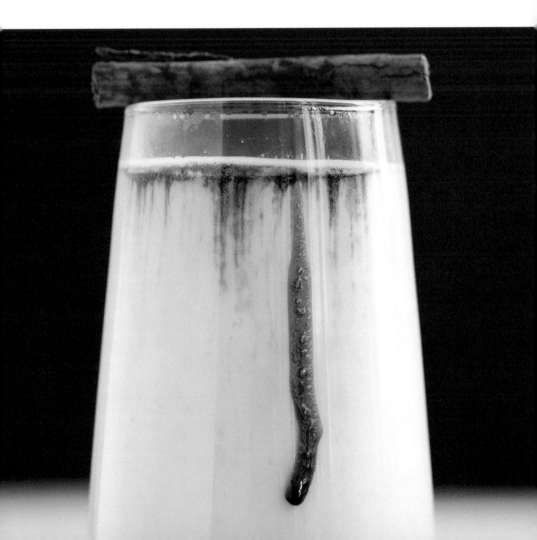

Chocolate mousse with chilli

- 1 large sweet potato
- 1 (200 g / 7 oz) bar of 85% cocoa dark chocolate
- 30 g / 1 oz butter
- Grated zest of ½ orange
- 1–2 tbsp. sherry or brandy (optional)
- ½ red chilli, very finely chopped (take care not to get chilli in your eyes!)
- 1 egg yolk
- 2 egg whites

Peel the potato and cut it into small chunks. Boil it in a little bit of water (just covering the bottom of the saucepan, so it's almost steamed). The trick is not to boil it for too long (it's ready when you can prick it without feeling resistance). You need 200 g / 7 oz mashed potato (use a blender, food processor or blender stick).

Melt the chocolate in a double boiler.

Add the butter to the hot chocolate and stir into the potato together with the alcohol (or orange juice), orange zest, egg yolk and chilli.

You can choose to stop here, leave it to cool in the fridge and eat it like nougat. You only need a little bit to bring colour to your cheeks and make your taste buds sing.

You can also get a lighter and more mousse-like consistency by beating a couple of egg whites and gently mixing them with the mousse before leaving it to cool. Delicious with a cup of hot tea without sugar.

This is a sensational dessert. You've never tasted anything like this before. I promise you! I've been inspired by a chef specialising in revolutionary seductive kitchen tricks for ladies in high heels!

Erotic fruit salad
Serves 2

- ½ fresh pineapple cut into small chunks
- Seeds of 1 pomegranate
- 1 banana, sliced
- 4–6 dates, finely sliced
- Coarsely chopped almonds that have soaked in water for at least 12 hours
- Coarsely grated or finely chopped 75% cocoa dark chocolate

- 1 cm vanilla pod
- ¼ tsp. ground nutmeg
- ¼ tsp. ground cloves
- 2 passion fruit

Toss the spices with the pineapple, banana, dates and pomegranate seeds.

Arrange on two plates and sprinkle with the grated chocolate. Scoop the contents of one passion fruit over each portion of fruit salad. Enjoy immediately.

Fruit and melon symphony to make your skin glow

- 1 cantaloupe melon, cut into bite-size chunks
- 1 handful black, seedless grapes, halved lengthwise
- 1 tbsp. balsamic vinegar
- 1 tbsp. lemon juice and zest of 1 lemon
- 1 tsp. freshly ground rose pepper (or crushed in a mortar)
- ¼ tsp. ground nutmeg
- ¼ tsp. star anise, finely ground (in an electric coffee grinder) or crushed in a mortar
- Salt flakes
- Fresh mint leaves for added flavour and decoration

Mix all the ingredients in a bowl and leave to soak for a couple of hours or, even better, overnight. Serve with a dollop of whipped cream if you want to be indulgent.

Carob delights
Serves 4

- 145 g / 1 cup almonds
- 4 tbsp. carob powder
- 35 g / ½ cup desiccated coconut
- 2 tbsp. pine nuts
- 2 tbsp. xylitol
- 50 ml / ¼ cup water or orange juice
- 200 g / 7 oz dates

Place all ingredients in a food processor and continue mixing until the dough forms a lump. You may need to add more liquid. Roll into balls and coat with carob powder, desiccated coconut and finely ground almonds.

Store in a tin, separated by baking paper. Keep for up to two weeks in the fridge. Enjoy them with a cup of liquorice chai, mint tea or green tea.

Pink grapefruit on a white cloud
Serves 2–4

- 2 pink grapefruit, peeled and all the white pith removed
- Seeds of 1 pomegranate, all the white pith removed
- Fresh rosemary leaves, approximately 20, coarsely chopped
- 1 tbsp. acacia honey
- 1 cm vanilla pod

A large dollop of plain soy yoghurt without added sugar, or Greek yoghurt sweetened with a little vanilla and xylitol.

Cut the grapefruit into chunks and place in a bowl with the pomegranate seeds.

Add the vanilla, honey and rosemary and leave to steep for a couple of hours (or several hours if you have the time).

Serve the yoghurt on a beautiful plate topped with the pink grapefruit. Decorate with rosemary.

Drinks

~~~~~~~~~~

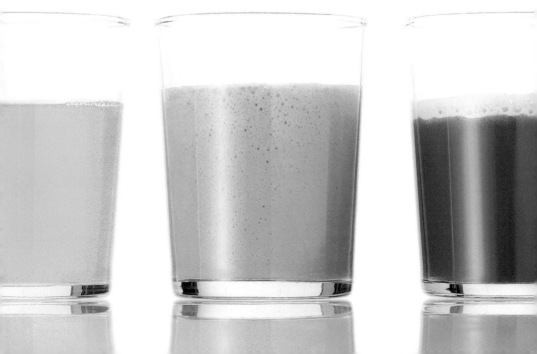

Green tea soft drink
Makes ½ litre / 1 pint

- 1 sachet Original Green Tea Powder. See www.pinetribe.com/thorbjorg/green-tea
- ½ litre / 1 pint soda water with lemon or lime

Empty a sachet of green tea powder into a jug. Pour the soda water into the jug, holding the jug at an angle, as the soda water will foam when it comes into contact with the tea powder. The foam settles within 10 minutes. You can try adding slices of orange or lemon, passion fruit, fresh ginger, a little honey or xylitol, ice cubes and mint leaves, apple peel or orange zest cut into spirals. Drink every day, throughout the day.

Variation: Green tea Mojito
Pour the green tea drink into tall glasses with plenty of fresh mint leaves and frozen melon balls (you can make these yourself). Sweeten with xylitol.

Hibiscus toddy
1 jug

- 15 g / ½ cup hibiscus flowers (from your local health food shop). Can be replaced by unsweetened cranberry or blueberry juice
- ½ litre / 1 pint water
- 1 cinnamon stick
- 30 g / 1 oz fresh ginger, finely sliced
- 200 ml / 1 cup pure apple juice
- Lemon juice to taste

Boil the hibiscus flowers for a couple of minutes in the water with cinnamon and ginger. Remove from the heat and leave to stand for an hour. Strain the liquid, heat the drink again and add the apple juice. Add lemon to taste.

Almond milk with mint

(The measurements for this drink work in proportions, so that you can make any quantity you like.)

- 1 part almonds (don't have to be blanched)
- 3 parts water
- 1 part soy or rice milk
- A suitable number of dates (4 dates per 70 g / ½ cup almonds)
- 1 cm vanilla pod
- 15 fresh mint leaves or a couple of dried mint leaves (mint tea)

Blend all ingredients in a blender with 1 part ice cubes. Enjoy immediately. You'll be in seventh heaven!

If your blender isn't powerful enough, your milk will be lumpy and you'll have to pass it through a sieve before drinking.

Delicious liquorice chai
Serves 2

- 300 ml / 1 ¼ cups mixed rice and almond milk
- 200 ml / 1 scant cup soy milk with vanilla
- 1 cm vanilla pod, cut lengthwise
- 1 cinnamon stick
- 4 tsp. whole cloves
- ½–1 tsp. liquorice root powder

Heat the milk with the other ingredients. Leave to stand for half an hour before reheating and drinking. Pour anything left over (including spices) into a thermos for later use.

If you would like to know more

~~~~~~~~~

See www.pinetribe.com/thorbjorg/inspiration

Club Vitality
Club Vitality is a hub for courses, tips, extra content and connecting with Thorbjörg. See www.pinetribe.com/thorbjorg/club-vitality

Books
See my recommendations and where you can get them on www.pinetribe.com/thorbjorg/books

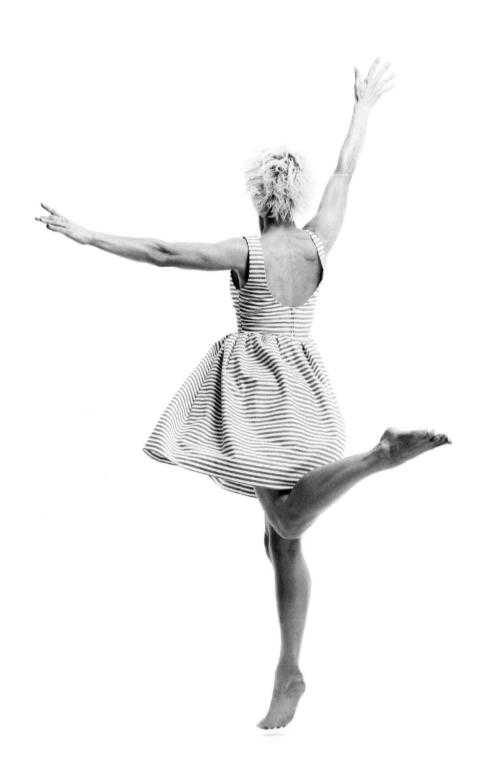

Bibliography

Harvard School of Public Health, www.hsph.harvard.edu/nutrition-source.

Harvard Nurses Study II.

Harvard Health Professionals Follow-up study.
Eat, Drink and Be Healthy 2nd Edition by Walter C. Willett (Free Press, 2005).

Loren Cordain, www.thepaleodiet.com.
The Paleo Diet by Loren Cordain (Wiley, 2002).

Professor Jennifer Brand-Miller, Sydney University, www.glycemicindex.com.

The Low GI Diet Revolution: The Definitive Science-Based Weight Loss Plan by Jennie Brand-Miller et al. (Marlowe & Company, 2005).

Professor Mark Houston, www.hypertensioninstitute.com.
What Your Doctor May Not Tell You About Hypertension by Mark C. Houston et. al. (Warner Books, 2004).

Bruce N. Ames, www.bruceames.org.

Liu, J. and Ames, B.N. (2005) Mitochondrial nutrients: Reducing mitochondrial decay to delay or treat cognitive dysfunction, Alzheimer's disease, and Parkinson's disease, In: Neurodegenerative Disorders, Aging and Antioxidants. Editors Y. Luo and L. Packer.

Ames, B.N. (2004) A Role for Supplements in Optimizing Health: The Metabolic Tune-Up. Arch Biochem Biophys., 423: 227–234.

Ames, B.N. (2004) Mitochondrial Decay, A Major Cause of Aging, Can Be Delayed. J. Alz. Dis., 6: 117–21.

Ames, B.N. (2004) Delaying the Mitochondrial Decay of Aging. Ann NY Acad Sci 1019: 406–411.

Ames, B.N. (2004) Supplements and Tuning Up Metabolism, J Nutr. 134:3164S–8S.

Ames, B. N., Elson-Schwab, I., and Silver, E. (2002) High-Dose Vitamins Stimulate Variant Enzymes with Decreased Coenzyme-Binding Affinity (Increased Km): Relevance to Genetic Disease and Polymorphisms. Am J. Clin. Nutr. 75, 616–658.

Ames, B. N. and Wakimoto, P. (2002): Are Vitamins and Mineral Deficiencies a Major Cancer Risk? Nat Rev Cancer 2002 Sep; 2 (9): 694–704.

Ludwig, D.S. (2003): Novel treatments for Obesity. Asia Pac J Clin Nutr 12 Suppl: S8.

Ludwig DS, Majzoub JA, Al-Zahrani A et al. High glycemic index foods, overeating, and obesity. Pediatrics [online] 1999;103:e26. URL: http://www.pediatrics.org.

Leibach, I et al. Morphine tolerance in genetically selected rats induced by chronically elevated saccharine intake; Science, 1983, 221 (Aug. 26): 871–73.

Leventahal et al. Selective actions of central mu and kappa opioid antagonists upon sucrose intake in sham fed rats. Brain Research 1995. 685 (July 10: 205–10).

INDEX

Lightning Source UK Ltd.
Milton Keynes UK
UKIC01n2204300414
230909UK00003B/9

9 780099 126092 8